I0526709

PHAT ACCEPTANCE

JESS MOWRY

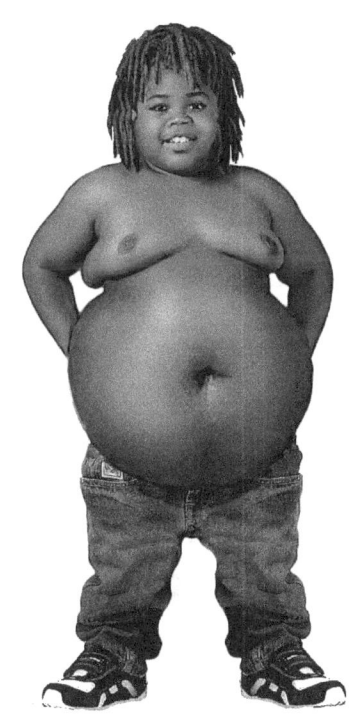

Copyright © 1997 - 2021 by Jess Mowry

PRINT ISBN-10: 0-9985579-2-7
PRINT ISBN-13: 978-0-9985579-2-2

EBOOK ISBN-10: 0-9980767-2-4
EBOOK ISBN-13: 978-0-9980767-2-0

First Anubis Edition 2016

ALL RIGHTS RESERVED - No part of this book or its entirety may be reproduced, distributed, or transmitted in any form or by any means, including photocopying, scanning, recording, or other electronic or mechanical methods, or by any information storage and retrieval system without the prior written consent of the author, except in the case of very brief quotations embodied in critical reviews and certain other noncommercial uses permitted by copyright law.

The scanning, uploading, and distribution of this book via the Internet, or by any other means, without the prior written consent of the author is illegal and punishable by law. Please purchase only authorized electronic editions and do not participate in or encourage electronic piracy – stealing - of copyrighted materials.

This is a work of fiction. Names, characters, businesses, products, places, events and incidents are either the manifestations of the author's imagination or are used in a fictitious context.

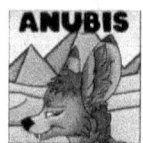

OTHER BOOKS BY JESS MOWRY

Rats In The Trees
Children Of The Night
Way Past Cool
Six Out Seven
Ghost Train
Babylon Boyz
Bones Become Flowers
Voodoo Dawgz
Skeleton Key
Tyger Tales
When All Goes Bright
Knights Crossing
The Bridge
Reaps
Drawing From Life
Ghost Ship
Midnight Sons
Magic Rats
Double Acting
The Coyote Valley Railroad
In The Dead Of Night
Spencer's Spirit
The Insiders
The Light

FOR ALL THE
PHAT KIDS

PHAT

ACCEPTANCE

Maybe he wasn't the world's fattest kid, but he *was* the fattest kid Brandon had seen! He wasn't the only fat kid in the house; of the thirty-two freshmen in History class at least eight were packing extra pounds from slightly chubby to triple-XL.

But this dude was off the fat grading scale!

Brandon tried not to stare at the boy, though he'd chosen a desk at the rear of the room *because* he wanted to watch everyone. His eighth grade Creative Writing teacher had said a good writer had to observe, but so far here on this first day of school, in these first few minutes of World History, there hadn't been a lot to observe that might have inspired a story. The kids were a typical Santa Cruz mix -- meaning that most of them were white -- from surfers in tank-tops, hoodies and baggies, to wiggers in big-jeans that showed-off their shorts. A pair of goths, boy and girl, had so many piercings that Brandon winced, although he wore an earring himself. There were also a couple of obvious jocks.

The surfers were tanned to the shade of old pennies. One could have starred in *Endless Summer*, a buff-bodied blondie with movie-star looks. Another resembled a wiry coyote, his body as hard as a sheet-metal roof in a 'beater that clung to a perfect six-pack and looked painted over the bricks of his chest; while a third was a rolly-

1

poly boy in a sort of charmingly baby-chub way with big bobby breasts and a soft swaggy belly, the latter lolling into his lap, who looked like he'd spent last night on a beach, with sand in his hair and beer on his breath.

The goths were as pale as vanilla ice cream and as bony as desiccated cadavers, while several boys were lazily lardy with most of their weight in their bellies and butts, their shapes suggesting eggs with legs from sitting and playing video games. One of the jocks could have been on TV as a model for All-American boys often depicted by Norman Rockwell... a sort of muscular Opy Taylor complete with freckles and rusty-red hair. There was also a skinhead in boots and suspenders who might have passed for an albino ape. About the only "statement" he made was that some Caucasians had lame-looking skulls and should have kept hair on top of them. Of the ten other white kids, Brandon included, most were fairly average in build... meaning that most looked a bit overfed compared to the 1970s kids that Brandon had seen in his mom's photo album. A couple of girls were "pleasingly plump," though another resembled a Barbie doll... which looked almost scary in real life.

In a front row desk sat a marshmallow dude whose belly spilled out from under his shirt, an Area 51 souvenir tee from the Little Alien Cafe. The shirt was at least two sizes too small and stretched over softly sagging boy-breasts, suggesting a sedentary summer of snacking at keyboard or game control, but cool in space-nerdy way.

The other students included three Asians; two slender girls who looked Vietnamese, and a Japanese boy either chubby or husky beneath a big tee with a red rising sun. Four kids were of Hispanic descent, and three of them undisputedly fat, a raven-haired girl with a friendly smile who embodied the term, "voluptuous," and a pair of dudes who bulged everywhere in white T-shirts and faded big-jeans. Two brown girls may have been Middle-eastern, their figures concealed by modest full dresses.

The black race hadn't been represented... until this ebony mountain of blubber had lumbered ponderously into the room.

That wasn't a good metaphor, thought Brandon; an author had to describe characters so readers could picture them clearly. For one

2

thing, mountains didn't "lumber." Nor did they quiver, ripple or jiggle, shimmy, shiver, or undulate... and this dude's body was doing it all. "Jell-O" may have been a cliché, but in this case it was personification. His chest was a pair of blatant balloons that looked about to burst from his shirt as they rolled, bobbled and bounced around, while his wobbly waist encircled his middle like some gigantic torus of flubber. His clothes were kind of carelessly cool; his T-shirt was black and at least 4-X, though it still couldn't cover twin pendulous masses composing almost the full lower half of an awesomely incredible belly that wallowed against his enormous thighs and plunged and rebound-ed with every slow step as if determined to touch-tag the floor; and he had to lean drastically backward to counterbalance their rippling bulk. Almost buried by all that loose lard and far overhung by the rolls of waist, were faded blue-jeans, their cuffs dragging the floor; and only the toes of his sneakers showed.

Brandon scrawled notes in his "writer's journal," a section reserved in his shiny new binder bought yesterday at the mall. At least this dude was something new, and a prime candidate for his Beast-world book, a graphic novel he planned to write as soon as he found an illustrator.

Brandon found he was staring again, not staying "detached" like a writer should be. He shifted his eyes from all that loose fat -- as deep, dusky black as a new truck tire and supported somehow on a boy's skeleton -- to study a face like an African cherub's. Opulent cheeks engulfed the dude's nose, which though bridgeless was wide at the tip and only looked small in that full-moon face... a very dark moon in this case. Still, his eyes, obsidian -- or maybe better described as onyx -- were anime large, and though not completely unguarded, suggested a pit-bull potentially friendly to anyone with the courage to pet him. His lips were full and expressive above two chins on a neckless neck, and were parted in sort of a pouty smile, revealing the gleam of fierce white teeth, which might have been his normal expression... like he just didn't *care* about being so fat, no matter how socially-incorrect, or what anybody might think.

The huge boy's hair was a lion's mane that tumbled over his

3

super-size shoulders to midway down his massive back, which was almost as rolly as his front. It might have been braided, or maybe dreadlocked, though Brandon wasn't sure about that, not being down with African Culture. He supposed it was only natural that the mammoth boy was waddling toward him, his vast belly clearing a road ahead as kids leaned aside to get out of its way.

The desks were arranged in five rows of six, with another four at the rear of the room, and Brandon sat in the back right corner, farthest away from the door. The desk to his left was still empty, while the rolly-poly surfer dude was somnolently sprawled in the third, smogging the air with alcohol fumes as well as an unabashed young male scent and shedding a virtual beach on the floor. Brandon had made a few notes about him, his ragged gray hoodie unzipped -- the sleeves had been brutally amputated -- casually baring the orbs of his chest and his lazily lolling pillow of belly, the latter spilling over the crotch of ancient cutoff Levis jeans; an old-school black-and-white sneaker untied – worn *sans* socks like its mate -- his hair a wild mop of salt-stiffened curls that sheepdog-like covered his eyes.

One of the white girls, an "average type," had taken the fourth desk beside the surfer but wasn't looking very stoked about her nearest neighbors. There was another empty desk in the first row at the front of the room, but any cool dude would have sat in the back and taken a chance on Brandon.

Brandon was cool enough, he supposed, though a little detached from the center of cool. If cool was a sun then he was a planet, not shining himself but reflecting the rays. At age fourteen he was five-foot-five, and a few careless pounds "overweight" in the belly -- if judged by current health-nazi standards -- with silky blond hair in a central part that flowed down over his chest and back like a feral young prince in a sorcery game. His eyes were dark blue, his nose pertly snubbed, and his lips rested partly open a lot displaying a pair of startling teeth that probably should have been tamed by tin. He had a few muscles in all the right places; his chest was high and gently defined, though his tummy gave him a Bugs Bunny look when his mind was involved with other things besides maintaining a physical pose. He'd tried working out with his big brother's weights

4

to buff up a bit for his high school debut, but had only developed a killer backache. A chiropractor had aligned his spine -- under the eyes of his worried mom -- while scolding him for being "brainwashed," and "falling for the movie-star image that Hollywood fed to American kids."

Still, Brandon managed to pose fairly cool; his tan was as deep as the drunk surfer-dude's, and he'd carefully chosen his wardrobe this morning to give him a sort of ambiguous look; a blue chambray shirt from his big brother's closet with three buttons open to show off his chest, along with a pair of loose Tommy jeans and experienced-looking Rocket Dog sneaks. Most Santa Cruz kids would have thought him a surfer -- hardcore skaters seldom had tummies -- and the drunk boy had dreamily greeted him, *duuuude;* a cool enough image to front in this town where everyone had to be something. It was also a look that didn't offend or attract much attention; good camouflage to be an observer without getting caught in anyone's mix.

The woolly black mammoth -- a good description, assuming mammoths had ever been fat -- was still on a cumbersome course for Brandon with every inch of his body in motion. Obsidian eyes queried Brandon's blue, confirming the empty desk wasn't taken. Brandon still fought to throttle his stare, but the dude was just so incredibly... **FAT!** Every step seemed like a separate struggle to further advance all his rippling mass; his gigantic thighs got in each other's way so he had to squeeze one in front of the other while sort of heaving himself side-to-side in the waddling gait of a ponderous penguin. Brandon glanced around again to observe the other kids' reactions.

The average white girl abandoned her desk, not wanting to sit with an unrated Brandon, a drunk and smelly surfer-dude, and now this enormous ebony beast... a word Brandon used as a compliment. She snatched her things and fled to the front, landing beside the "51 kid," who nervously tugged at his undersized shirt then crossed his arms to conceal his boy-breasts... which of course only drew attention to them.

The other two surfers were smirking at the sight of the mammoth

5

boy fighting to walk. The All-American looked disgusted in a requisite jock-brained way. The skinhead was beaming a stupid hate stare -- though of course it wasn't based on weight -- that he probably practiced every morning while scraping the fuzz off his simian skull, while the 51 kid seemed a little relieved at no longer being the fattest in class. The Latino dudes appeared impressed, while the Japanese boy was scanning the black as if maybe thinking of Sumo. A few of the students were looking confused, as if not knowing how to react: fat kids were common enough in their world -- even if not *this* extreme -- but there weren't many black kids in Santa Cruz and nobody knew much about them. Their movies and music were ass-kickin' cool; and Brandon had heard all the usual stories about how strong and bad they were: but this dude didn't fit into that role any more than his clothes fit him.

Then, Brandon wondered how *he* should react? The other students were watching him, too, since he seemed to be the black mammoth's objective – did they think they knew each other? He felt as if he was up on a stage and no one had told him what part to play. This enormous fat boy was invading his space on the very first day of *high school*, dammit! It felt like his cool was a house of cards and this huge black beast was shaking the floor.

Brandon had gone to a private school from kindergarten through eighth grade so he didn't know anyone here. He had no posse to take his back and validate his coolness permit. He remembered something his father had said about making career decisions. Nobody would dis him for dissing this dude, but they'd probably dis him for not. And they'd have him under a microscope for all this freakin' period. *Observer, hell!* he told himself; *he* was the one who was being observed... scanned, filed, and categorized, labeled and tagged for the next four years by how he treated this fat black kid in the space of the next few minutes!

He turned for support to the sandy surfer, who sprawled with sockless sneaks splayed out in silver puddles of sand. He was wearing a charm around his neck, a little wooden tiki god suspended on a leather strip between the lolling spheres of his chest, their nipples inverted like soft little slits. His eyes were still hidden beneath his hair, a messy mop of tangled locks bleached by years of sun and salt. A rat was tattooed on one of his arms above a chub-padded bicep; a Disney kind of cartoon rat who grinned around a big cigar, the sort of thing a kid would love but most adults would hate. Words were tattooed underneath -- Tola Rats, whatever that meant -- but, any dude who had a tat would naturally be cool, and his judgment would be weighty in this Freshman student court.

But, dammit, he was sleeping!

The mammoth black boy had finally arrived. The effort of walking – to term it as such -- had gleamingly sheened him with silvery sweat, darkened the shirt beneath huge upper arms -- which were bigger around than Brandon's thighs -- and painted it over the orbs of his chest, which bulged as big as flubber-filled melons. His vast body seemed to radiate heat, like being close to the steam locomotive that chugged though the Santa Cruz Mountains. Brandon almost expected a hiss of air-brakes as the dude came puffing to a halt, though his body continued to wobble for several seconds afterward. His scent was strong and blatantly male, though Brandon wouldn't have called it bad; and he found himself a little surprised that the boy wasn't any taller than he, though at least four times the diameter.

The dude wiggled out of his ancient pack -- one of those no-name K-Mart kind -- his shirt climbing up over acres of belly, his navel a tunnel into blackness between those pendulous teardrops of fat, and which could have easily swallowed an orange. Sweat dribbled out to spatter the floor; and again Brandon thought of the steam locomotive, which always seemed to be leaking. Those jeans weren't actually doing much to cover the dude's enormous bottom, which looked like a pair of black planets colliding. He seemed... well, just too fat to wear clothes, like something never *meant* to wear clothes; huge, black, steamy, slow, yet somehow suggesting enormous power.

It was also strangely embarrassing to be so close to the boy's mammoth body, especially now with that belly thrust out, its soft midnight mass almost pulsing with life, feeling his heat, steamed in his scent, with everyone else observing. It occurred to Brandon that, huge as he was – at least on the horizontal plane – the dude was

7

probably only fourteen and could have found a larger shirt to "decently" cover his social shame. Brandon turned to the surfer-boy, still hoping for a backup; but the dude was lost in space somewhere, or maybe riding waves. Brandon felt betrayed somehow, as if he'd been sentenced without a trial by a jury who wanted an execution and his public defender was out to lunch, yet there was nothing he could do but smile and say, "What's up?"

Total silence ruled the room. Every ear was listening. The place was like a pack of raptors massing for attack. ...But, could the prey defend itself? The dude didn't look like a video thug, but his size was still intimidating; a locomotive loose in the room. What could it do? Slam you aside if you got in its way? Smash you under its awesome weight? Should it be respected, rejected, or feared?

Snickers were stored away for the moment, and smirks were carefully traded. Insults waited locked and loaded, but who would be the first to fire?

The goths looked understanding. The jocks just looked disgusted as their roles required. The skinhead chewed on broken glass and didn't seem to like the taste. The brown boys traded Latin glances cryptic to Caucasians; and the Anglos seemed to realize that four of them were "overweight"... and one of those a surfer.

"Chillin'," said the black dude in a husky voice like a kid with a cold, though maybe because of his roll-padded neck. "S'up with you?"

"...Oh. ...Phat," said Brandon, the first "black thing" that came to mind. As soon as it was out of his mouth he felt his cheeks flash red. "I mean with a P," he added, sweating. "You know? Like, phat is cool?"

He almost expected a crushing "duh," which might have turned the raptors on him, but the huge boy only chuckled. "I heard you, man."

TWO

Then the bell rang and the teacher came in. The other kids turned like Pavlov's dogs as if expecting Scoobie Snacks... but they would *remember* that Brandon had smiled and spoken first to the huge fat dude. The incredible boy sat down in the desk, and Brandon watched in fascination.

The boy almost had to put the desk *on*, like donning a personal spacecraft. This took a lot of puffing and struggle and rearranging of rippling rolls; and Brandon actually held his breath, wanting to help but not knowing how. He remembered an ancient classic cartoon of an overloaded Arabian camel whose legs had splayed in four directions beneath an impossible burden. He expected the desk to do the same and dump the huge kid on the floor. But somehow the thing held together despite many ominous creaks and squeaks, and the boy finally managed to squeeze into place, though the desk would be altered forever. Most of his midnight middle was bare, avalanching over his thighs where the seams of his jeans were splitting, as well as the moons of his gigantic bottom, while his breast balloons rolled on the desk top, and Brandon wondered how he could write. It was lucky that no one had seen the show: the kids were watching the teacher now, and probably scanning for weaknesses.

The teacher, Mr. Rosenberg, had seemingly chosen not to watch and might have distracted the class on purpose by squeakily chalking his name on the board.

Brandon scribbled "careless fat" on an empty page of his journal. It seemed like an apt description; a dude so fat he just didn't care that his body overflowed his clothes and steamed the air around him. A locomotive might be cool, a puffing, massive, midnight thing, but

9

careless of its awesome size so you approached it carefully. He turn-ed to the boy and whispered: "Um? Are you okay?" Then his cheeks got red again: had he just said something else uncool?

The fat boy only flashed his smile. "Guess I can wait fifty minutes to breathe. Figured the desks would be bigger in high school."

"Yeah," agreed Brandon. "Would've thought so, huh? ...Um, do you need anything from your pack?" It was clear the boy couldn't reach it... there was way too much of him to reach over.

The dude studied Brandon a moment. "Sure, man. Snag me a pen and the binder."

Brandon flicked a glance at the teacher, who'd turned from the board and was facing down eyes. He looked somewhere in his mid-dle forties and obviously knew about animal taming. He also acted pretty cool, not seeming to notice when Brandon got up to get the fat boy's things. The binder was ancient and battered, but covered with wicked graffiti cartoons of Bambi-eyed black boys in various poses. Many were shirtless and several were fat, their oversize jeans sagging comically low. The dude offered Brandon a chubby hand, displaying dimples instead of knuckles. "Thanks, I'm Travis."

Brandon was guided through twists and turns in one of those complicated shakes. He'd never touched black skin before... *what a stupid thing to think!* Like, what was it going to do, rub off?

"Brandon," said Brandon. "Um, did you draw all this stuff?" he added, indicating the binder. "Those 'toons are crazy cool."

"Yeah. Thanks, man," the huge boy replied. "Just a little thing I do."

Mr. Rosenberg cleared his throat, and Brandon scuttled back to his desk. A couple of kids looked over their shoulders, but no one seemed very interested now. The teacher flipped open a folder and smiled. "Good morning, ladies and gentlemen, and welcome to World History. Which, believe it or not, you're a part of."

The skinhead raised his hand. "Are we gonna learn about Aryans? Or just that multicultural crap?"

The jocks and surfers snickered, but with him or *at* him was hard to tell. The 51 kid seemed a little embarrassed, maybe for the sins of his race, while the brown boys scowled at one-another but otherwise didn't react. Brandon scanned for Travis's view, but the fat boy only looked amused, as if a baby had cooed the F-word.

Mr. Rosenberg's smile didn't change. "This is *World* History, Mr...?"

"Uh, Slater," said the skinhead.

"Joe Slater?"

"Yeah. It's an Aryan name."

"Anglo-Saxon, actually. A mender of roofs... slates, you know?" Mr. Rosenberg marked the roll. "Unfortunately, we live in a country that doesn't spend much on education. We have many new privatized prisons, and are building more every year. We also spend billions on various wars, but we don't have the funding for 'frills' in our schools, such as music, art, and up-to-date books. Or a special class for Euro-pean History. However, I think you ought to know there never was an Aryan race. If you want to study Aryans, you'll need to focus on languages... and at your own expense."

The skinhead's skull flushed neon pink. "That's a... not true! I got a book!" He frantically dug in his pack.

"Ah, yes, I'm familiar with *that* one. And, of course, *The Iron Dream*... another one of your favorites, I'm sure. I've also read *Mein Kampb*... as you've probably tried to. However, Mr. Slater, it's either true, or else there have been many other books written... by *genuine* scholars... for the sole purpose of deceiving you. But, I'll be happy to give extra credit for a well-researched paper on Aryans."

Some of the kids looked curious. Joe just looked confused.

Mr. Rosenberg scanned his folder. "Please answer up as I call your names. And correct me if I mispronounce."

"Woah," whispered Brandon to Travis. "I didn't know that, about Aryans."

Travis nodded. "Never were any, just a language. Want me to wake up your homie?"

"Um... sure," said Brandon. This didn't seem like the time to explain he didn't know the surfer.

Travis's desk creaked painfully as he leaned way over his massive middle and tapped the surfer's shoulder. The dude woke up and shook back his hair, scattering sand like a silica blizzard. "Huh?" His eyes were blue, anime large, and widened even more. "Woah!" he breathed. "Are you ever *fat!*"

He didn't say it loudly, but it drew a few snickers here and there. Also a frown from the teacher.

"You ain't no bone-bag yourself," observed Travis, rather matter-of-factly.

The surfer scanned his surroundings, seeming surprised to wake up in school. He could have still been half-asleep, or maybe still more than slightly drunk, but he had a dreamy kind of face and might have always looked that way. His teeth were big and beaver-like, and his hair tumbled over his eyes once more so only his puggy nose showed, giving the sheepdog impression again. Then he smiled and slapped his belly, which jiggled like the Jell-O cliché. "Dude! We're brothers!"

Travis smiled. "I think I know what you did last summer."

"Yeah, heh," said the boy. "Been totally heliotropic, man. Best summer I ever had in my life!" He searched the sandy floor at his feet. "Aw, beans! Musta left my stuff at the beach!"

"Um," whispered Brandon, trying to see around Travis's bulk and feeling a little left out. "I've got an extra pen. And tons of pape..." He suddenly became aware that silence ruled the room again, and Mr. Rosenberg was frowning.

"I have a 'Bosco Donatello' penciled into my class." He regarded the roll a bit dubiously as if someone had added that name as a joke. "Where might this gentleman be? ...Or not?"

"Oh, heh," said the surf-boy. "Yo, teacher-dude."

A few kids promptly snickered, but the other surfers looked surprised and turned to stare at Bosco.

"Thank you... dude," the teacher replied and went on reading names. "Travis White" also got snickers, being an oxymoron, but "Brandon Williams" got nothing, not being ethnic or anything odd, though he was Estonian on his mother's side.

Well, thought Brandon, at least one of his teachers was cool this year. But he had to survive the rest of the day, sort of like mapping a minefield. He'd almost stepped on a mine already, but surfer Bosco had saved his butt, had taken his back by talking to Travis.

Mr. Rosenberg closed the folder and roamed the room with his eyes. "I seldom alter seating arrangements... unless there's an obvious problem... but I hope it won't be a case of 'Why Are All The Black Kids Sitting Together In the Cafeteria.' That would be history repeating itself, and those who don't learn from history are always doomed to repeat it."

Brandon felt embarrassed for Travis, as if the teacher had singled him out, but Travis only smiled.

"Mr. Tanaka?" added the teacher, turning to the Japanese boy. "Would you please pass out the texts?" He glanced at a stack of books on his desk and frowned at their aged and battered condition. "Such as they are."

The next few minutes were normal enough for a first day of school anywhere, Mr. Rosenberg sketching the course while Tiger Tanaka distributed books that looked as if they'd been through a war. If someone had snickered at Tiger's name, Brandon had missed it while talking to Travis. He slipped from his desk to give Bosco some paper and one of his extra Pilot pens. Bosco thought the pen was "boss," like something he'd never seen before, and started drawing a rat on a surfboard, and not without considerable skill. Mr. Rosenberg noticed Brandon but seemed to approve of his charity.

"You surf, dude?" asked Bosco. "You got the look."

"Nah," said Brandon. "But I hang at Santa Cruz Beach a lot. And I usually skate every day."

"Skurfs are cool," said Bosco. "Got one myself."

"...Skurfs?" asked Brandon.

"You know? Skurfboards. ...Sidewalk surfin'?"

"...Oh yeah. My dad said they used to be called that back in the 1960s."

"You oughta check out real surfin', dude. Ain't nothin' so boss in the whole universe! Not even sex, heh. ...'Less it's havin' it in the ocean."

Brandon considered that picture, then shrugged. "I'm probably too old to learn."

"Nah, man. Anybody can. I could teach you easy. 'Specially if you ride a skurf. Them things are treacherous, woah! They skid all over

13

the place!"

"What kind of wheels do you ride?" asked Brandon.

"The regular kind." Bosco circled a finger and thumb. "You know? About this big."

"...Oh," said Brandon. "But, surfing looks really hard."

"Nah," said Bosco. "Cement, *that's* hard. Like, bust your buns. Heh." He turned to Travis. "How 'bout you, big black kahuna?"

Brandon winced but Travis chuckled. "I can float really good."

"Um?" asked Brandon. "Does it ever bother you, being so black?"

"Huh?" asked Travis and Bosco together.

Brandon's cheeks flashed red again. "I... mean fat," he stammered, which though in retrospect still a *faux pas*, was at least a state of being capable of alteration.

Travis smiled. "Somebody's Freudian slip is showing."

"Huh?" said Bosco.

"Sorry," said Brandon.

"I've always been fat," said Travis, and didn't sound bothered about it."

"Bet you always been black, too," said Bosco, making Brandon wince again, but chuckled and went on: "You'd be a natural long-boarder, Travvy. I got some big old beauties at home just dyin' to meet a dude like you."

"I never heard of black surfers," said Travis, then glanced at Brandon. "Or fat ones either."

"Then you never been to Hawaii," said Bosco. "They got some *huge* kahunas there! An' it wasn't white people invented surfin'."

"Food for thought," said Travis.

"Cool tat, Bosco," offered Brandon.

"Thanks, dude. Got it when I was eight. ...Oh, an' thanks for the paper, too." Bosco searched his hoodie pockets. "Aw, beans! I don't got my schedule! It's back on the beach with my stuff. ...I guess."

"Beans," agreed Brandon, intrigued by this new synonym for shit, cool in an understated way.

"Can I borrow yours, Brandy-buck?"

"...Um... I need it myself. I don't even know where the rooms are yet."

14

"Well... could you copy it down for me?"

"Planet earth calling," said Travis. "It's Brandon's schedule, Bosco-dude. What good's it gonna do you?"

"...Oh yeah."

"What are your classes?" asked Brandon.

Bosco shook more sand from his hair as if creating his personal beach. "...Well... The regular kind, I guess. ...Like, um, History..."

"We're in History," said Brandon.

"Oh yeah."

"Yo," said Travis. "Ask if you can go to the office and get another schedule."

"Gentlemen and dudes," said the teacher, materializing suddenly. "I'm glad to see the races and..." He glanced at Bosco. "Other species mingling. But, I must ask the question; do we have a problem?"

"Oh, heh," said Bosco. "No prob at all, Mr... um...?"

"It's on the blackboard, Mr. Donatello."

"Oh yeah. I can see it from here."

"Um," said Brandon. "He lost his schedule."

"I'm sure it's wherever his mind is. ...Come up to my desk, Mr. Donatello. I'll give you a pass to the office."

"Woah," said Bosco after the teacher walked away. "He's kinda cool, huh?"

"Yeah," said Travis. "And your ass is lucky."

Bosco got up, swaying dangerously, and Brandon grabbed his shoulders.

"Heh," said Bosco, blowing beer fumes in Brandon's face. "Guess I'm still kinda buzzed. Can't remember nothin' last night."

"Did you have sex in the ocean?" asked Travis.

"I think I woulda remembered that."

"Well, pull up your pants if you don't wanna brag."

"Oh. Heh. These are my lucky cutoffs. But, they got kinda small this summer."

"Now we know you're a natural blond. ...Funny, you don't look Italian."

"A lot of Northern Italians are blond, but I get asked that a lot."

"Learn something new every day," said Travis.

15

Bosco ambled away, boy-breasts bobbing bouncily – Brandon hastily scribbled -- and belly lapping over his jeans like the cheerfully lolling tongue of a puppy, while shedding more silver sand on the floor as if he was scattering stardust. The other surfers flashed hang-loose signs, which Bosco returned with a careless smile.

"He's kind of a mess," ventured Brandon. "But, a cool kind of mess."

"He could sink the *Titanic*," said Travis.

Brandon smiled. "Was that a Freudian slip?"

"Sometimes a cigar is just a cigar."

THREE

The rest of first period was pretty routine for a first day of school on planet earth – or at least in the U.S.A. -- the kids mostly trying to housebreak their minds after three months of letting them go anywhere. The teacher established his rating of cool by not assigning homework that day, except to "look over the book tonight"... which naturally nobody would. The office was right across the hall, but Bosco got lost and was gone half an hour.

"You could have followed your trail," chuckled Travis, dragging the toe of his sneak through the sand as Bosco finally plopped down at his desk.

"Oh, yeah. Heh."

"Did you sleep on a beach last night?" asked Brandon.

"Oh yeah," sighed Bosco dreamily. "Ain't nothin' so boss in the whole universe than wakin' up to the sound of waves an' the sun shinin' rosy an' gold on the water." He closed his eyes as if seeing a picture. "Like, God just finished makin' the world an' you're the first dude who gets to see it. ...Like bein' born all over again."

Brandon made a note of that, surprised Bosco could be poetic. Then the bell sounded out in the hall, and most of the kids had leaped to their feet before its last echo had died. Brandon suddenly realized he'd made two friends in these first fifty minutes, but now he'd have to go it alone in five more alien atmospheres. He quickly shouldered his Sideout pack, not wanting to leave but scared of a tardy. "Maybe we can hook-up for lunch?"

"One of my favorite subjects," said Travis. "Despite being stereotypical."

17

"See ya there, Brandy an' Travvy," said Bosco.

Panic and urgency curdled the air as Brandon hurried into the hall. Kids crowded past in a jostling herd, the younger ones looking bewildered. Brandon felt like a fool with a map in his hand, and it wasn't much comfort to see other Freshmen scanning their maps with desperate expressions while slammed aside by older kids who knew their way around. There were curses and various threats, as if Freshmen were an inferior race that nobody wanted to integrate, though Brandon had been prepared for that, thanks to his older brother. But, this was the safest school in town, with only four shootings and one homicide to blemish its record last year.

Just like back in history class, most of the kids were white. Brown was the next predominant color, the other majority Asian. A few black students flowed along or battled against the teenage tide like night-colored salmon fighting upstream. A white dude pushed Brandon and called him a queer, but Brandon ignored him and kept on going. Other bullies lurked by lockers like bears on a riverbank waiting for fish. Brandon got spit on once or twice, was called a number of nasty names -- none of them new and improved -- and hit in the face with a wad of gum... which wasn't as bad as he'd expected. He finally found the freakin' "quad," and his second class was near the front in another building across a lawn. He blinked in the bright September sun, catching the salty scent of the sea a mile away in Capitola, and reached his room with minutes to spare. There were a lot of empty desks, but Tiger Tanaka was already seated, his binder open, a pen in hand like a stereotypical smart Asian kid.

This was a class that Brandon had wanted, one of his two electives, but he stopped outside to catch his breath and observe the rowdy stream of teens. A lot of the dudes were showing skin, their shirts unbuttoned carelessly, though never accidentally. Brandon unbutton-ed his own all the way, revealing his dangerous Tommy jeans and several inches of blue Calvin shorts.

"Hey, dork!"

Brandon turned as a boy approached, worming his way through the bustling bodies. "Yo, Troy. Wuttup?"

Brandon Williams and Troy Durrant had met each other when

both were five. They had cruised their skates a million miles and always dreamed of surfing someday. They had shared a lot of their Wonder Years and had a thousand adventures together, like getting drunk at ten years old and passing out on Santa Cruz Beach. They had finally awakened just after dark to find their shoes and shirts were gone! Also Brandon's Tommy jeans, leaving him only tightey-whities. Then they had seen a Latino boy who seemed to be wearing Brandon's gear, and had chased him across an acre of sand and brought him down like a pair of lions, ripping off his jeans and shirt - - like trying to skin a tiger alive -- before realizing those *weren't* Brandon's clothes! Luckily, Troy still had some cash, and the kid was persuaded to sell his things... after they'd chilled him out a bit.

But this summer hadn't been the same: Troy had gotten a surf-board, but had also developed what seemed like a fetish for pumping iron and body-building... which Brandon found terminally boring. Troy did look cool with his new definition; but Brandon got tired of watching him "work" while having to make admiring comments and feel him up like a sweaty pony in some perverted petting zoo. The gain of Troy's summer was now on display in a tight T-shirt and loose jean-shorts. His hair was buzzed and golden-brown, his eyes a brilliant indigo. His face was Caucasian perfection without even a ghost of a zit, though looking confused at the moment.

"Where the hell's World History, man? This mookin' map is retarded!"

Brandon took a casual pose and leaned against a locker. "Chill out, dawg. I'll hook you up."

Troy cocked his head. "Who you been hangin' with... 'homie?'" Then he laughed. "You look like Shaun in The Partridge Family with all that 1970s hair. Don't make a *total* fool of yourself, especially on the first day of school. *I* know you're a dork, but nobody else does... yet."

"Thanks, I needed that." Brandon pointed to the quad. "World History's in front of that building, right across from the office. And the teacher's cool, didn't give homework."

Troy looked relieved. "Thanks. The fat old cow in English class is givin' it out with a bullet! *Tale Of Two Cities*, first chapter tonight!"

19

"Been there, done that," said Brandon. "Back in seventh grade. ...'It was the best of times, it was the worst of times.'"

"You should have stayed in private school." Troy glanced around at the swarming students. "Compared to these losers you're already Harvard. ...Speaking of which, can you help with my homework tonight?"

"When have I not, challenged one?"

"Sucks we only got P.E. together."

"You can beat me at hoops as usual."

"Have to do that in your driveway tonight; it's football season, remember?"

Brandon groaned. "I hate football!"

"This isn't your preppy school, dork; you don't have a choice what to do in P.E."

"It wasn't a prep school, ferret face. But, that ostensibly sucks."

Troy punched Brandon's shoulder. "Welcome to public education, where everything ostensibly sucks."

"Can't you see your counselor and switch to one of my electives?"

Troy laughed. "You think these counselors actually counsel? And writing's your thing, I can't write shit." Then he gave Brandon a scoping. "You should have gotten in shape this summer. Used my weights and buffed your bod. Your tummy looks like a pot-bellied kid's. Suck it in, twat... no, wait, leave it out."

"Huh?" said Brandon. "Like, make up your very small mind."

"Girls, dweeb! Three o'clock. You make me look ostensibly good."

Two girls went by, and not in a hurry. One was blond, tanned and cute, in a T-shirt, jeans, and big leather sandals. Brandon felt like he'd seen her before but couldn't remember where. She seemed to give him the ghost of a glance, and maybe a spook of a smile.

Then a black dude sauntered past, maybe fourteen and buff as a brick. He was clad in big-jeans at maximum sag, while a wife-beater clung like a coat of paint to six-pack abs and high-jutting pecs. Brandon gave Troy a nudge. "Deflate, little guy, he's out of your league by at least a light-year."

"It's natural with *them,*" muttered Troy, gazing after the midnight god. "You check his pecs? ...Way out to *here!*"

"Yeah cool, but I don't wanna marry him."

"I gotta get a shirt like that!"

"It's not the shirt, boy-wonder, it's what it can't hide that reveals the inside."

Troy pulled up his shirt. "How do I look?"

"I assume you want some stroking, and hopefully only the verbal kind since we're out in public?"

Troy gazed after the black boy again. "And it's natural with them!"

"You said that already."

"Did you check out the blond babe checking me out?"

"I think she was checking me."

"In your dreams!"

"May they all be wet."

"Hey, Brandy-buck."

"...Oh. S'up, Bosco?" Brandon asked, as the rolly-poly surfer appeared. "Sure aren't those lucky cutoffs."

"Oh. Heh." Bosco gave his jeans a tug, and Brandon noted that, like Travis's, the rear belt loop was broken from always being pulled. ...It was one of those details writers observed.

Bosco held out his schedule. "You know where this is? I'm all confused."

Brandon's eyebrows arched. "You have Creative Writing?"

"Guess so. Heh. They got my records all skeezed up. Like, I ain't on their I.B.M. or somethin'. So, I got two electives that wasn't full."

"Well, this is one of them," said Brandon. "But we still have a couple minutes."

"I better go in. I'll save you a seat. I'm totally lost in space today."

Troy had been staring at Bosco. "Shit!" he said after Bosco left. "You know who that is?"

"Bosco Donatello, unless he's incognito."

"You retard! That's *the* Bosco Donatello! He was on the cover of *Pipeline*, man! The Endless Summer special in June. Don't you ever read anything except those infantile fantasy books?"

"He was in Pipe?"

"On the freakin' *cover*, ass! He won that big Hawaiian thing. The

Pacific Surfing Championship."

"He said he'd been to Hawaii." Brandon glanced into the classroom, where Bosco now sprawled in a desk. "You sure that's him?"

Troy snorted. "You sure you're not a retarded zombie? He's the only fat kid I ever saw with his picture on a magazine cover, except for anti-obesity stuff."

"I'd call him more chubby than fat."

"On whose rating scale?" Troy jerked his jaw toward a Latino boy, one of the pair from History class. "'Chubby' compared to that tub of lard?"

"Shut up, dork!" hissed Brandon.

Troy only shrugged. "He probably doesn't speak English."

"Hey, Troy, you're really a mook sometimes. Ever hear of hate speech?"

"Hey," said Troy. "People can't help being other colors, but nobody has to be obese."

"Nobody has to hate, either."

"What's that supposed to mean?"

"Like, who the mook died and made you God? Like, to judge anybody? ...But, I guess they don't judge surfing skills by how much somebody weighs."

Troy glanced through the doorway at Bosco. "He'd look cool if he lost fifty pounds. Maybe he can surf like a star, but he'll never get a movie deal or do any ads or commercials unless he loses all that fat."

"He doesn't seem sad about it."

"You know him now?"

"Not in the biblical sense. Want me to get you his autograph?"

"Mook, yeah! ...Wish I had that magazine. He could sign the cover to me. ...You got any other classes with him? I'll call mom and get her to bring it. Maybe we can meet him at lunch."

"I already met him, and we're doing lunch, dude."

"Cool!" Troy looked up at the hallway clock. "But I only got two minutes. How the mook can I call her now?"

Brandon reached into a pocket. "You can use this if you kiss my ass."

22

"Looks too much like your face. ...You got a new phone?"

"Mom's idea," said Brandon. "This one has a panic button direct to 911 so I'll be 'safe' in public school."

Troy snatched the phone, but then his eyes narrowed in sudden disgust. "Shit, Brandon! Check *that* out!"

"Yo, Brandon," said Travis, lumbering up like an earthquake in Jell-O, puffing like a steam locomotive, and sweating like an ebony pony who'd galloped ten miles though a desert.

Ignoring Troy, who stupidly stood with the phone to his ear, Brandon smiled and offered a hand. Travis gave him the shake again, so fast it looked like Brandon knew it. "Bro, you lost?" asked Brandon.

"Nah, man, I never get lost. Always got my course laid out. Shortest distance between two points. You have Creative Writing, too?"

Brandon was surprised... a black kid taking a writing class? "Sorry, I could have come with you, like, taken your back on the way."

Travis laughed. "I'm way too fat to get shoved. Besides, I shove back. And I'm black so I might have a gun."

"Bosco has this class, too. He's already inside."

"Surprised he didn't get lost again."

Troy stepped away to plead with his mom.

"We should check our schedules," said Brandon. "See what else we have together."

"P.E. next period?" asked Travis.

"Yeah. ...And Health and Science in fourth after lunch."

"And Math in sixth."

"Oh," said Brandon. "This is Troy, who's calling his mom. Troy, this is Travis."

"S'up, man?" said Travis.

Troy barely nodded. "Not much."

"Bosco's saving a seat," said Brandon.

"I'll save you one," said Travis.

Troy tossed the phone to Brandon after Travis left. "She's bringing it."

"Is she pissed?" asked Brandon.

23

"She'll get over it. She's picking me up after school anyhow. Dentist appointment. ...Who the hell was that black blubber tub?"

"Long-boarder star."

"You can't be serious! He'd need one as big as a garbage barge!"

"Actually he's a Beastworld prince. Panther genes, of course."

Troy made a face. "That's totally disgusting! He's so fat he can hardly walk! His parents should be put in jail for letting him get so freakin' fat! There's an obesity epidemic!"

"That's a stupid thing to say 'cause 'obesity' isn't catching so it can't be epidemic. But I guess it's supposed to scare me as much as terrorism."

"Maybe it is terrorism," said Troy. "Like, how can America protect itself if kids get too fat to join the Army?"

"Then we couldn't make wars for oil."

Troy scowled. "We couldn't fight sand-niggers, either."

"Watch your mookin' mouth, fool! Or *you're* gonna need protection!" Brandon quickly glanced around, noting several chubby dudes, but no one black or Middle-Eastern.

Troy shook his head. "Why are you always defending fatties?"

"The mook are you talking about? ...Because I don't like you dissing people?"

"Obese people *should* be dissed."

"Haters should," said Brandon. "But I've taken your back a few times. Like when you got jumped on the beach for dissing a fat little kid. ...With two big brothers defending him."

"Aw, they were Vallies. Fat-ass Vallies."

"Who almost put you on your skinny ass."

"Hey, I'm not skinny!"

Brandon shrugged. "I've got one fat friend... and maybe I made two more today. And you're right, I'll defend them from haters, so don't be one, okay?"

Troy glanced into the classroom again, where Travis was struggling to put on a desk. "Obese people shouldn't have friends. Being rejected might make them lose weight."

"You're really a mook sometimes."

"You said that already. ...And aren't you getting a little too old for

24

role-playing games anymore? I do my surfing for real these days."

Brandon laughed. "Graduate from the grommets yet? Or, still riding down at the sewer plant?"

Troy looked at the clock. "See you at lunch. ...*With* Donatello!" Bells went off along the hall. "Shit! I'm late!"

"I'm not. See?" Brandon stepped casually into the classroom as Troy took off at the speed of light.

FOUR

Brandon had been prepared for P.E. like a going to a dentist... expecting to suffer in various ways but still hoping to come out alive. He definitely wasn't a wussy, with muscles, a tan, and a few basic moves, but he'd never liked organized sports or dealing with grown-ups who forced kids to "play."

His private school had given kids choices as if they really had minds of their own and should be encouraged to use them. Soccer had been a popular game, along with Greek Dodge or basketball if you wanted to be on a team, but there was also a swimming pool, and kids could use the computer lab, or spend recess in the library if they didn't feel up for physical stuff.

He wasn't shy about dressing down; he'd been stripping for gym in sixth-grade, while most public schools didn't make kids get naked until a year or so later. He wasn't a nudist or anything weird, but his mother had always professed a belief that human bodies were natural things so baring them wasn't a sin or a crime, and the family had gone to the Free Beach a lot when Brandon and his brother were little. He still swam naked at home, along with his brother and Troy, so being bare-assed among other bare asses wasn't anything new.

Except now he was one of the smaller asses.

In second period he'd been surprised to find his Writing teacher was black. But, Mr. Akida had six published novels along with a couple of story collections -- and by mainstream publishers -- which made him mega-qualified. Mr. Akida was thirty-something, slenderly built and dark-chocolate-skinned, with sable braids that swept his shoulders. He'd asked the class if they'd done any writing during

26

their summer vacation, and most of the kids had looked confused... was this some sort of sneaky test?

But, Brandon had passed in a trio of stories about the adventures of two mutant boys who'd escaped from a secret laboratory. They'd been injected with animal genes -- those of lions and tigers from Earth combined with beasts from other dimensions -- as part of an evil experiment to spawn a race of worker slaves. The story took place on Beastworld, a mostly uninhabited planet of sunny blue oceans and tropical islands. The project hadn't been going well: some of the beast-boys were turning out wild instead of submissive... like the pair who'd escaped from the Beastmaster's lab. These were the heroes, Bucky and Beast, and their quest was to bring down the evil Beastmaster and set all the mutant kids free. The stories were part of a graphic novel; the book that Brandon planned to write as soon as he found an illustrator.

Tiger Tanaka had turned in a tale, though Asians were always smart: but Travis had also brought a story, surprising Brandon even more. Some of the kids had taken the course in hopes of getting an easy A, while a few, like Bosco, had only been added to fill an empty desk. Travis, Tiger and Brandon were the only ones who'd written that summer, except for a chubby girl who wrote poems. A few of the dudes had smirked at them as if they'd done something nerdy; but Bosco had managed to stay awake, and had even made a few notes... on Brandon's paper with Brandon's pen.

It had seemed like an inspiring class, and Brandon was still elevated by that as he waited in front of the gym. Then a whistle blew and somebody roared in a voice like the evil Beastmaster's.

Brandon's brother had warned him that Coach Dinklehoff was a moronic goon with hair everywhere except on his head... and hadn't exaggerated much. The boys were bellowed into the gym, a vast and echoing cavern that reeked of sweat and sour old socks while broiling under mercury lights on a day that was already hot. Boys began to lose their shirts, and Brandon unbuttoned his own. The coach bulled his way to the bleachers, mounted to pose like Mussolini, flipped open a clipboard and slavered out names.

The boys were ranked alphabetically, putting Brandon in a back row with Travis, while Bosco was forced to the front of the lines to stand with Troy Durrant. Brandon was amused to see that Troy was too shy to talk to Bosco, obviously awed by his reputation despite dissing him for his fat.

Also in front was the muscled black boy who Troy and Brandon had seen in the hall. He nodded to Travis as if they were friends, which Brandon supposed was natural... the only black kids in the house. The dude looked like an anatomy model with every tight muscle starkly defined; and Troy kept giving him envious glances, obviously wanting to take off his shirt, but bashful at being so underdeveloped compared to the African god. The black dude didn't seem to care about the awesome shape he was in: his posture was appallingly sloppy, his six-pack belly thrust carelessly out, while his paving stone pecs would have sagged if they could; and he only peeled off his snowy wife-beater when the heat of the lights and the bodies around him had risen to nearly volcanic extremes.

Brandon murmured to Travis, "I guess Bosco's locker won't be near ours."

Another boy gave him a smile. "Your homie can trade with somebody."

If Travis White was the world's fattest kid, this dude rated a close second-place, his belly pouring out of his shirt and hanging halfway to his knees. Brandon had tagged him as a Latino -- old-penny copper with long raven hair -- but his name was Danny Little-Wing.

"Yeah," said Danny, when Brandon asked the logical question. "I crack whenever I see those stickers on somebody's Beamer or SUV. 'Native Californian,' my ass!"

Brandon's mother had one on her Saab. "Are you a Senior?" he asked.

"I freakin' wish," said Danny. "Then I'd be out of this suckhole next year. Just a lowly Sophomore, dude."

"Former buffalo soldier," said Travis, reaching past Brandon to shake Danny's hand; and Brandon felt like a skinny third-grader squished between the two mammoth boys.

Danny shrugged an enormous shoulder. "Guess it wasn't your idea to help the white man slaughter the red man. There used to be a bounty on us; twenty bucks a head... dead."

Travis smiled. "I won't bore you with the slavery thing."

"Um," said Brandon, trying to breathe. "I didn't do it. But, I know I benefitted from it."

Travis chuckled. "That's more than most white people admit."

"It's a start, anyway," said Danny, stepping back a pace, allowing Brandon some atmosphere. "Sorry, man. I don't even know where I stop anymore and the rest of the world begins."

Coach blew a saliva-spray blast on his whistle. "Shut up back there! ...Oh. Little-Wing. You want the Special Eds this period? It's extra credit and you can use it."

Snickers rippled the ranks of boys: everyone knew that "Special" wasn't.

"Sure. Why not?" said Danny. "I've even got opposable thumbs."

Coach snapped his clipboard shut like a bite. "Line up for your locker assignments! Through that door over there! And everyone dresses down! And you *will* take showers today! ... You! What?"

Bosco had his hand up. "Coach dude," he said. "I can't dress down."

"You're not *that* fat!" bellowed the coach, as if Bosco didn't have *much* leprosy, drawing a few more snickers and laughs as the other boys bustled away.

"Huh?" said Bosco. "Nah. I mean, like I can't 'cause..."

"Don't be a little *girl!*" roared Coach as if that was the ultimate insult to any adolescent male.

And it was a stupid thing to say, considering Bosco's hoodie was open, proudly displaying his boy-breasts and belly; but Brandon had noticed a couple of kids -- the marshmallow dude in the 51 shirt, and another boy standing beside him -- who were looking a little scared. It was like they had known this moment would come, but maybe they'd hoped for a pardon? The other boy wasn't chubby or fat: he looked normal enough, though young for high school.

"Huh?" said Bosco again. "Nah. Hey, coach dude. Like, what happened is..."

"Listen up!" bellowed Coach, ignoring Bosco. "Special Eds! See Little Wing! Over there in the red T-shirt!"

29

Somebody laughed. "Red tee-pee, more like it!"

Most of the boys were already in line at the double doors to the locker room -- Troy gave Brandon a hurry-up wave -- leaving Danny, Travis, and seven others alone in the sweltering gym. Four boys were fat to different degrees -- disregarding Danny and Travis -- the Latino boy from History class, the boy in the Area 51 shirt, and chubby Bosco Donatello. There was also a boy in a grimy old tee that might have been urban camouflage... or may have once been white. He seemed to have swallowed a basketball, though he wasn't fat anywhere else. Beside him stood the little dude, who looked eleven and ready to cry; and also the muscular ebony boy. Brandon had lingered with Travis -- the line was in alphabetical order so he had plenty of time -- and Bosco came ambling over.

"Is Coach a skeeze, or what?" he grumbled. "I was only tryin' to tell the trog I left my gym clothes at the beach."

Danny Little-Wing laughed. "They got loaners. But I hope you've had all your shots." He studied Bosco and smiled. "Boys with innies can ride the wind."

Bosco looked down at his chest. "Huh?"

"My grandfather told me that," said Danny, patting his own enormous orbs. "I got 'em, too. But, you don't have to be Special. You're not fat enough to be obese."

"What's obese?" asked Bosco, as if he'd never heard the word.

"Dangerously overweight," said Brandon, before he thought about it.

The brown boy gave him a glare. "Dangerous to who?" he demanded. Then he stepped to Brandon. "The hell you doin' here, skinny-ass?" He studied Brandon and narrowed his eyes. "Don't I know you from somewhere?"

Brandon was more surprised than scared – he'd been called many things but never skinny -- and studied the boy in return. The dude looked a little familiar, and it wasn't from History class. He also noticed a gang tattoo across the dude's chubby knuckles. "I... don't think so, man."

"'Chubby compared to that tub of lard? ...Probably doesn't speak English?' That ring any bells in your head, *amigo?*"

30

FIVE

"Oh," said Brandon. "But, hey, man, *I* didn't say that."

Danny stepped to the brown boy. "Peace-out, bro. I'm large an' in charge."

"Yeah," added Travis, putting a hand on Brandon's shoulder. "An' this's my dawg."

"Wuttup?" asked the muscular black dude, ambling over to stand with Travis. He straightened his sloppy posture a bit like a lazy panther coming alert.

"My cousin Kelvin," said Travis to Brandon.

"Hey," said Brandon, taking the boy's offered hand and doing the shake Travis had taught him.

"Wait a minute," the brown boy said. "I *do* know you!"

Brandon checked the dude's face again... and suddenly saw it smaller and younger snarling at him in the dark. It was the boy from Santa Cruz Beach... the kid who Brandon and Troy had skinned!

"...Oh," said Brandon. "I... um, still got those Tommys we bought from you."

The dude cocked his head for a moment, then looked down and jiggled his belly, which avalanched over his jeans. "I don't think they fit me no more. Besides, you paid for 'em, man." Then he laughed. "An' twice what they was worth."

"I'm really sorry about that," said Brandon.

"Guess we all look alike to you, huh?"

"No, man, I got my clothes stolen. I told you after."

The boy snorted. "Yeah, after. ...Hey, man! You got any clue what that felt like? Getting' chased by you guys in the dark an' havin' my clothes ripped off?"

31

"...I guess not too cool."

"Like, what you think I was thinkin', man? I thought you were gonna rape me or somethin'. An' it had to be one of *us*, huh? Like, white dudes wouldn't have rolled you, huh?"

"I'm sorry, man. What else can I say?"

The boy shrugged. "Aw. That was four years ago." He smiled. "An' it was kinda funny. ...After. I'm Carlos."

"Brandon," said Brandon, shaking the boy's gang-tatted hand.

Travis was looking curious, but Bosco asked, "How do I get obese?"

Everyone cracked... except the Area 51 kid. The small boy had edged to Brandon's side, maybe to offer more backup. He didn't look "Special" to Brandon -- curly brown hair, an elf-like face, steel-rim Harry Potter glasses, and the convex curve of a little-kid tummy enhanced by a childish sway-back posture -- though way too young for high school. His Pokémon T-shirt hung down past his knees and made him look even smaller.

A wiry boy came trotting up with a battered clipboard and a tarnished brass whistle. "Coach said to give you these, Danny." He looked around at the other boys. "P.E. sucks! Wish I was Special."

"Hey, Ralph," said Danny. "So, get fat and hang with us."

"I wish, but the 'rents would kill me."

"Anybody want a whistle?" asked Danny. When no one answered he tossed it away stone-skipping over the floor. "Don't need no stinkin' whistles." He turned to Bosco again. "'Obese' is the latest hate-speak. Like nigger, beaner, honkey... or wop. It's something haters and health-nazis call you." He pointed to the locker room doors where the other boys were filing through. "There's a dude who's fatter than you, but only a hater would call him obese."

"I'm obese," said the 51 kid.

Danny gave him a thoughtful look. "Only if you wanna be."

"I think I'm just fat," said Bosco. "There's nothin' dangerous about me."

"I'd call you chubby," said Brandon. "If I had to describe you by weight."

"Me too," said the boy in the camouflage tee, whose belly seemed

32

to be seeking escape.

Brandon gave him a scoping... maybe that *was* a basketball under his tightly straining shirt? The dude's skater jeans were years out of date -- Skunks with black-and-white stripes down the sides -- and he wore them so low that his sneaks were hidden beneath their ragged tumble of cuffs. His hair was a mop of rusty-red straw above a sort of tough urchin face liberally dusted with freckles, and his eyes were as green as a cat's. "Hey, man," said Brandon. "I've seen you down at the Boardwalk."

Carlos laughed. "Did he jack a pair of your Tommys, too?"

"Give it a funeral," said Brandon. He faced the basketball-bellied boy. "You work at Captain Softee Cone. Killer chocolate dip."

"Yeah," said the boy. He grinned, and grasped his spherical tummy as if preparing to make a shot. "I'm quality-control."

"I must have bought a hundred from you. They totally rock," said Brandon.

"We got that much in common," said Carlos.

"No offense," said the pot-bellied boy. "But a lotta dudes look like you at the beach."

"Tell me about it," said Carlos. "Can't tell one blond from another."

The pot-bellied boy was studying Brandon. "I kinda remember your hair. ...Oh yeah, you're Tommy's bud. I'm Zach."

"Brandon," said Brandon, shaking hands.

"What's all this Tommy stuff?" asked Danny.

"A friend of mine, not the jeans," said Brandon.

"Yo, Zach," said Travis. "My folks got Neptune's Fish 'N Chips. Under the coaster by Corn Dog Cavern."

"Oh yeah," said Zach. "Best fish 'n chips on the 'walk, man. But I'm down at the other end between Pelican Pizza an' Buccaneer Burger."

"Your joint kicks ass," said Carlos to Travis. He slapped his belly, making it ripple. "This ain't all burrito blubber."

"You work at the Boardwalk, too?" asked Travis.

"Nah. But, I hang there a lot. My dad's a mechanic, fixes the rides. An' mom works in the nurse's office."

"Sorry, Zach," said Danny. "You're not fat enough to be obese. Surfer-dude is borderline on the fat-hater scale, but even Coach wouldn't call you obese. An' it's football season, so he needs a few heavyweight orcs."

"I got asthma," said Zach.

"Yeah? How bad?"

"How bad does it gotta be?"

Danny smiled. "Sounds bad enough." He scribbled something on the clipboard. "Bring me a note tomorrow... an' make it look like it's from a doctor." Then he faced the elf boy. "What's your dysfunction, little big man?"

The kid looked down at his huge puppy feet encased in sneaks like cartoon kicks. "I'm just... little."

The other boys had moved together like a convention of meet-and-greet bellies... except for the 51 kid. "Okay," said Danny. "But you're gonna need a note for somethin'. An' it can't just be for bein' little."

"Like what?" the little dude asked.

"Asthma?" suggested Zach.

"Too many kids got asthma," said Danny. "Try bronchitis, it's easy to fake. Just cough like you're gonna spew whenever Coach is around."

"Cool," said the boy. "How do you spell it?"

"I'll write it down, bring me a note... and make it look like it's from a doctor."

"No prob."

"What's your name?" asked Travis.

"Rex."

"Yo, T-Rex." Travis shook hands with the little dude.

"How old are you, man?" asked Kelvin.

"Thirteen. I skipped eighth grade."

Danny turned to Kelvin. "*You're* gonna need a major excuse if you wanna be a Special!"

"I gots a heart problem," said Kelvin, his posture gone sloppy again. "I ain't supposed to run."

Travis added, "He'll bring you a real doctor's note."

"Um?" asked Brandon. "How did you get all those muscles, Kelvin? A friend of mine worked out all summer but he never got as ripped as you."

Kelvin shrugged. "Come with the package, I guess."

"He eats like a garbage-disposal," said Travis. "Laziest dude on the planet, too."

The 51 kid spoke again: "Do Specials have get naked?"

"It's part of the P.E. ritual," said Danny. "Making kids get naked seems to fulfill some deep adult need."

"But, I'm obese and I hate it."

"Hey," said Travis. "You're with your brothers. I show you 'obese' with a bullet!" He wriggled out of his shirt and fat seemed avalanche everywhere in a rippling, rolly midnight cascade.

"That's my cuz," said Kelvin, leaning on Travis's shoulder.

Everybody looked awed. As Brandon had already noted, Travis was really too fat to wear clothes, and now without them -- or nearly so -- looked more like some ebony mutant beast-boy grown to heroic proportions. The rolls of his waist were so enormous, and his belly hung down so far in front that his jeans were secured around his thighs by a punker studded leather belt that had to have come from a Big and Tall store. His gigantic bottom was more than half bare, and his boy-breasts were massive midnight melons, their nipples the size of soda can tops but stretched out smooth so they didn't protrude and almost matching the rest of his color. He grinned at Brandon. "My eyes are up here, but no charge for admiration."

Brandon blushed, but Bosco laughed. "How much for coppin' a feel?"

"Buy me flowers and candy, with emphasis on candy."

"Woah, you're *awesome*!" exclaimed Rex in obvious unabashed admiration.

"I can't get naked!" howled the 51 kid. "I don't want people to see I'm obese!"

"You really *are* obese," said Travis. "The most dangerous kind, which is in your mind. What's your name? ...Though I don't think I care."

"Jason Gray. I'm on a diet. In a month or so I'll be normal."

"I went on a diet once," said Danny. "But I'm back to normal now."

"What's wrong with you, Jason dude?" asked Bosco.

"I told you! I'm obese!"

Danny frowned. "I think we shall tire of that word fairly soon."

"Hey, Jason," said Brandon. "Everyone puts on little weight over summer vacation." He patted his tummy. "See? I did."

"I know I did," laughed Zach.

"I should have gotten active," whined Jason. "And dieted more. My mom's always telling me to."

"Then it's your fault you're obese," said Danny. Then he added a little more kindly, "Trade lockers with someone an' shower with us." He smiled. "Down in the Pig Pen. We got your back. Like Travis said, we're brothers here."

"...Well," said Jason. "Maybe until I lose some weight."

Rex laughed. "I'll take it, I sure as hell need it!"

Brandon glanced to the locker room doorway: the line was getting shorter. He wasn't sure why he said the next thing; maybe because he liked these dudes. He pictured them all together, laughing and getting to know each other while he had to play a stupid game. ...Yet, it seemed deeper than that; all his life he'd done what he wanted, gone where he wanted, been who he wanted, but here was something he couldn't do just because of his weight. ...Or, actually, the lack of it. "So, what does it take to be Special?" he asked.

"Bein' obese, I guess," said Bosco.

Jason flared, "Why would you wanna be obese? You think it's funny or something?"

"I'm starting to think you're funny," said Brandon.

"Try asthma," said Zach.

"Or bronchitis," said Rex.

"It can't be anything major," said Danny. "Then you'd be Physically Challenged. There's a separate class and a teacher for that."

Brandon considered. "What about a back problem?"

"You have one?"

"I used to. And it might flare up."

"You'll need a note. Make it look real." Danny wrote Brandon's

36

name on the clipboard. "Bosco, you'll need a note, too."

"What should be wrong with me?" asked Bosco.

Brandon laughed. "You have an allergic reaction to anal-retentive morons."

Bosco grinned. "What he said."

"How about epileptic?" said Danny.

"Like havin' spaz attacks?"

"How about cataleptic?" said Brandon. "That means you fall asleep a lot and don't know where you are."

Bosco grinned like a beaver. "That's me."

Danny wrote on the clipboard. "Those kinds of things are good 'cause Coach doesn't know what they mean. Welcome to the blubber club."

"So, what do we do?" asked Bosco.

"Walk laps, what else," said Danny. "Unless it's raining. Then we sit on the bleachers in here and watch the skinnies play B-ball. Or sometimes old sports movies. We saw *Field Of Dreams* six times last winter. Think you can handle that much pressure?"

"Do we have to take off our shirts?" asked Jason.

Everyone groaned. Zach stripped out of his camouflage tee, revealing a pale bulging spheroid of belly distended awkwardly over his jeans, striped with red longitudes of stretch marks and quivering like a bulbous balloon inflated to the edge of explosion, though his chest was fairly muscular.

"Wicked!" said Rex. "How long did it take you to get like that?"

Zack proudly patted himself. "Three months of dippin' softee cones an' eatin' all the rejects."

"How do you mook-up a softee?" asked Brandon.

"It's hard but I practice."

"My mom looked like that for a while," said Carlos. "Before she had my little sister."

Brandon stripped off his shirt, displaying his Bugs Bunny tummy, which wasn't very impressive. Then Rex pulled off his tent-like tee, revealing a featureless little-boy body as pink and white as a Caucasian baby's. He turned to Jason. "Lose it!" he ordered. "Or everybody will think you're a puss!"

"Or worse," said Danny, "a little girl."

"That's not fair!" cried Jason."

"Yo, Jason," said Carlos, losing his shirt to display bulging boy-breasts and rolls of brown blubber, his navel a smile upside-down. "In a month you won't have to hang with us. You gonna get skinny, remember?"

"Um?" said Brandon to Danny. "How does the grading system work? I'm trying to maintain a B-plus average."

Danny smiled. "I'm goin' to college, too. Learn the ways of the white man an' take back California."

"You can take it back from us," said Carlos. "After we take it back."

"It's mostly up to me," said Danny. "Walk laps on the track and you'll get a B-plus." He glanced at Jason. "Don't lose your shirt and I'll give you a D. Don't take showers, and you'll get an F. ...A big obese F."

"Do Specials ever get A's?" asked Rex. "I gotta overachieve."

"It's theoretically possible, but Coach hates giving A's to fat kids. He calls it rewarding failure. You could volunteer for towel-boy, but in your case I wouldn't advise it. No offense, but you're too cute."

"I have that problem, too."

"You could be our runner. Your mission, should you choose to accept it, is foxing off to the candy machines and keeping everybody supplied."

"I can do that. Nobody notices me anyway."

Jason said, "I'm not supposed to eat candy."

Danny rolled his eyes. "Nobody's gonna make you."

"But, if I don't will you give me an F?"

Danny glanced at Brandon. "You're right, he is funny... in a sad sort of way."

"And obese," added Zach.

"Yo, Danny?" asked Travis. "What about the swimming pool? I need to work on my tan."

"I need to start," said snowy-white Rex.

Carlos groaned. "Why is havin' a tan so cool, unless you was born with one?"

Danny shook his head. "That's only for the swim team. Besides, there's no supervision."

"Oh yeah," said Travis. "Like *we're* gonna sink?"

Danny shrugged. "Fat kids aren't supposed to have fun. It seems to fulfill some deep hater need."

SIX

The afternoon air was sticky and hot, a steamy stew of seashore scents, as Brandon, who'd lost his shirt at the bus stop, came up the heat-shimmered sidewalk and paused in front of his house. The ocean lay glassy across the street below the thirty-foot sandstone cliffs, emerald-green along the shore and shading to indigo at the horizon. The swells were nothing but slow-rolling humps, stirring the beds of golden kelp as they undulated over the reefs. The sky was clear and cloudless; the sea lions out on their own little rock seemed too sleepy to bark; and even the seagulls were lost in space, nodding in rows on the white wooden rails that lined this part of West Cliff Drive.

An occasional ruddy-faced middle-aged jogger plodded along the asphalt path that followed the edge of the cliffs. They looked out of place in this slumbering scene, panting, puffing, pouring sweat, as if running from something that rode on their shoulders and clung to their flesh with gargoyle claws. Maybe, thought Brandon poetically, they were trying to run away from *time*, as if they thought they couldn't be caught as long as they kept running.

A dozen surfers were out off the Point beyond the sea lion rock. Of course there weren't any waves right now, but they were still astride their boards in a place where nothing could catch them. Maybe not even time. Some had their suits peeled down to their waists; and Brandon pictured armored knights at rest upon their battle steeds.

Another world he would never be part of.

He studied the somnolent sunlit scene and tried to recall the savage sea that crashed and roared in winter storms, hurling waves

40

against the cliffs and flinging spray across the street that rattled his window glass. It seemed like a different universe now.

Or maybe another time.

The sleepy smell of summer lawns mingled with the seminal sea, and flowers bloomed along the block in brick-lined beds and red-wood borders, adding sweetness to the mix like breathing cotton-candy fumes. A mower grazed the grass next door in Tommy Turner's big front yard. Its driver was an almost bare boy with shaggy chocolate-colored hair and skin as tan as Brandon's, clad only in short, ragged cutoff jeans. He was twelve with big brown eyes and a chubby chip-munk face like Theodore without the fur. His body was mostly made of rolls beginning on top with a rolly chin that rolled on a roll around his neck, then rolls of fat rolling under his arms, which were also rolly. His chest was a pair of bobby balloons that jutted somehow aggres-sively and quivered and jiggled and bobbled about as the mower cruised the lawn, while rolling upon another roll that rolled upon a rolly belly that rolled way over his rolly thighs below the rolly roll of his waist. His cutoffs looked more like a decoration than any attempt to clothe himself since his vast bubble bottom was bare on the seat and just as tan as the rest of him.

Brandon scanned his own front lawn... he should have mowed it yesterday. Tommy saw him, grinned and waved, shifted gears, raised the blades, and drove the mower up the walk. The John Deere could have plowed a farm, shiny green and dangerous, the baddest mower on the block and all the neighbors knew it. Tommy cut the engine and sleepy silence settled.

"What's up, Brandon?"

Brandon let his tummy out: he'd kept sucked while walking home... as if the neighbors gave a shit about his BMI. "Dudes with innies can ride the wind."

Tommy switched off his I-pod and pulled the buds from his ears. "Zot?"

"An Indian dude said that today."

"Did he have innies, too?"

"Yeah. And so does another dude."

Tommy cupped one of his breasts in a hand and regarded its soft

41

innie nipple, which like Bosco's, Brandon had noted, was almost indiscernible from the rest of his coppery coloration. "They're crazy cool. ...You sure he was an Indian?"

"His name is Danny Little-Wing, sounds authentic to me."

"What tribe?" asked Tommy.

"Said he was an Ohlone."

"I read about them in fourth-grade," said Tommy. "This used to be their land around here, but I thought they were extinct."

"Guess the strong survived."

"Is he fat?"

"With a bullet!" Brandon spread his arms.

"Cool. A lot of Indians are. There's a dude in Arizona who saw our site last week. He's thirteen and a Papago, and they get mookin' *huge!*" Tommy spread his own arms wide. "We traded pics last night." He pulled a bottle from a holder. "Here, cool off a little. It's hotter than Beastworld with both suns out."

"Thanks," said Brandon. "But Diet Coke gives me headaches."

"Same here," said Tommy. "But it's real Coke on the under."

Brandon took a long, sweet swig and gave the bottle back. "Your mom got you on *another* diet?"

Tommy made a pukey face. "This one's based on grapefruit... retch! I been ordering dinner from Mobile Meals." He slapped his belly, making it wobble, his navel an oval-shaped cave into shadow. "I always gain weight on her diets... three pounds this week since she started to starve me."

"You'd think she would figure that out."

"She just finds it perplexing." Tommy drank some Coke and blasted a burp. "But I think she's starting to get a glimmer that diets don't work on me." He laughed. "'Specially since I have breakfast with you, lunch at school, hit McDonalds on my way home, and order Mobile Meals at night."

"Are you gaining weight on purpose?" asked Brandon. "Like, to get revenge on her?"

"Not anymore, but I used to." Tommy grinned. "You mean you never noticed? I'd eat everything in your house."

"When did you stop doing that?"

42

"Bite me, Bucky. Da Beast need lots of energy to mobilize all his fabulous fat."

Brandon studied Tommy. "Speaking of which, you got a lot fatter this summer, huh?"

"You never noticed that either? Almost twenty pounds." Tommy hoisted his belly blubber, revealing the fly of his cutoffs open and the tip of his shaft pertly peeking between the plump squeeze of thighs. "Can't even button 'em no more."

"Well, I see you every day."

"I know what you mean," said Tommy, releasing an avalanche of fat to cascade over his lap. "It's the reverse of seeing your grandma at Christmas, and all of a sudden she got really old." He studied Brandon's tummy. "You put on some weight yourself. Looks cool on ya, Bucky."

Brandon glanced down. "My old jeans were getting tight. These are bigger, another inch."

Tommy reached to Brandon's jeans and tugged them down a little more. "If you love your fat, set it free. It's the cool fat look, unbuttoned, unzipped."

Brandon smiled, regarding himself. "Some people would say it's only cool if you don't have to look that way. Like being born with a tan."

"Speaking of which," laughed Tommy, "I got another offer today. People drive by and see me mowing and think I'm a Mexican kid. I oughta start a business." He patted the side of the tractor. "She'll do almost ten on the street. I could drive anywhere in town. Rode her to McDee's yesterday."

"You sure got brown this summer," said Brandon. "But, why would you wanna work? You get a zombie-killer allowance."

Tommy frowned. "Mom cut it down to forty a week. She thinks I'm spending it all on food. Like, I don't have other needs on my socieo-economic level."

Brandon looked down at his tummy again. "Guess I did gain a little. But, hey, it was summertime. And I had a big lunch at school so it's sticking out if I let it."

"Why wouldn't you let it? Feels good being stuffed."

"Yeah, sort of careless," said Brandon. "And the food was actually edible."

"Yeah? What was it?"

"Burgers, burritos. Tamale pie. Pizza, meatloaf and other cool stuff. They have some deadly desserts, too; pies, cakes, and ice cream."

"*You* ate all that for lunch?" said Tommy. "That's my kinda happy meal."

"'Course I didn't eat all that. I was kickin' with some other dudes and saw what they were having. ...Um, so how do you feel, Tommy?"

"About the meaning of life, the universe and everything? I give it a 42."

"Being fat, duh."

"Me Da Beast!" Tommy suddenly leaped from the tractor and launched his bulk upon Brandon, crashing Brandon down on the lawn and pinning him on his back. "How does that feel, Bucky-boy?"

"Hey!" gasped Brandon. "C'mon, get off! I can't breathe under you!"

Tommy sat up on Brandon's chest as if astride a surfboard, his belly bulging in Brandon's face. "Is Da Beast cool?"

"Yeah, the coolest. Now get off."

"Does Da Beast rule on Beastworld?"

"Yeah! Will you get off me, man!"

"If you kiss my big fat belly."

"Bucky knows Da Beast's one weakness!"

"Okay! Don't tickle, I'll wet myself!" Tommy started to roll off, but Brandon grasped his belly, shaping it into a blubbery ball and sud-denly broke out laughing.

Tommy cocked his head. "What's funny?"

"I think I got it."

"My belly?" said Tommy. "Play with it all you want, no charge."

"I mean the symbolism."

"Oh that," said Tommy. "Yeah, it's very Freudian."

"Like, yours is bigger than mine."

"And now it's in your face."

"Or just hanging out," said Brandon. "Like, from under some-

44

body's shirt. Like it's too big to be contained. And the way some fat dudes walk, leaning way back with it thrusting out. Kinda aggressive."

"And/or threatening," said Tommy. "Though a lot of Freud's theories have been discredited."

Brandon added, recalling Danny Little-Wing and being squeezed between him and Travis, "Or bumping or pressing against you. *That's* why I felt embarrassed today, a couple of times. And your moobs are kind of aggressive, too."

"Thanks," said Tommy, puffing his chest more aggressively. "But moobs sounds crude. And as an acronym for 'man-boobs,' implies that boys *have* boobs, which infringes upon the rights of girls." He gath-ered his quivery orbs in both hands. "I prefer the term, boy-breasts. ...As to fat being aggressive, it's mostly a subconscious perception, and it disturbs a lot of fat-haters." He rolled off Brandon and got to his feet, leaning way back to balance his belly, his back bowed into a drastic curve, and tugged his cutoffs up a little below the wobbly rolls of his waist, though the moons of his bottom were still mostly bare.

Brandon sucked air. "I never knew you weighed so much."

Tommy laughed. "Back when I was little and didn't wanna do something, I just sat down on the floor. No way could mom get me up. Also quite effective for embarrassing her at the mall until offered a placating snack."

"I believe it," puffed Brandon. "Makes me think of Sitting Bull. He must have been an awesome dude to get a name like that."

"Huh?"

"Like, picture a sitting bull."

"...Oh, yeah."

"So, how are you paying Mobile Meals if you only get forty a week now? That's barely enough for two of their dinners."

"Plastic of course," said Tommy, leaning against the tractor. "Mom's got so many she can't keep track, and a new card comes in the mail every week at a low introductory interest rate." He snagged the bottle and gulped some Coke then offered it to Brandon. "I meet the van out here at the curb so mom don't know I'm getting

45

supplied."

Brandon drank the last of the soda, then pillowed his head on his arms. "You're bitchin', Beast."

"You'd bitch too if your mom was trying to starve you."

"No, it's an expression; a descriptive adjective. Means you're really cool."

"Never heard it before," said Tommy.

"You're boss, too."

"Mookin' right! Bitchin' and boss. That's me all over." Tommy happily fondled his fat. "And there's a lot of boss bitchin' me."

"But don't you get dissed?"

Tommy laughed. "Twenty-four-seven in this universe. But, you oughta know that already. Or don't you listen when we go out? 'Specially with no shirts."

"Guess I just tune it out," said Brandon. "Haters say shit to me, too. Like, homo, hippie, and... retch... golfer."

"I don't listen either," said Tommy. "You gotta accept that mooks gotta hate and *they're* the ones mooked-up, not you. Or you'd do a school massacre."

"So, how was your first day of school this year?"

"No massacres so far."

"Any other fat kids there?"

Tommy plopped down on the grass beside Brandon like a junior Sitting Bull. "With all this new health-nazi shit a lot of 'em are only chubby, but they have a sorta *controlled* look, like the Beastmaster's brain-wiped slaves. Like, set 'em free an' they'd get fat and look as bitchin' as me. But some are still cool. You can always tell a cool fat dude by how he wears his jeans."

"I noticed that today. I call it the careless look. The mookie dudes try to wear 'em way up. Like over their bellies not under them. Sorta like old golfers."

"Yeah, that's a major mookie."

"How about cool fat girls?"

Tommy smiled. "Lots of fat girls are smart, which is like a bonus."

"What about P.E.?"

"Usual mookshit, walking laps. Like, that's gonna make fat kids lose weight. That's as stupid as TV commercials to 'go out and play for an hour every day.'" Tommy gave Brandon a thoughtful look. "We never talked about fat before."

"Is that cool?"

"It's about mookin' time! I've only been fat for twelve years." Tommy jiggled his blubber again. "And I'm the phattest kind of fat, like Mexican kids and Indians, real soft and rolly."

"Yeah," said Brandon. "I guess if you're gonna be fat, you should be the phattest kind."

"Def," agreed Tommy. "'Course, if you're just starting to get fat, like during summer vacation, it mostly goes to your belly first. I call it the basketball look."

"Like Zach at the Boardwalk?"

"I didn't know you knew Zach."

"He's in my P.E. class this year. But, we bought a million cones from him. He remembered you."

"I usually go and hang with him when you and Troy are doing stuff. He lets me run the place sometimes. I'm boss at dipping softees."

"Ever mook 'em up?"

"It's hard to mook a softee."

Brandon sighed. "Seems like all I've been doing with Troy this summer is watching him lift his mookin' weights."

"That's gotta be zombie-boring."

"Even to a zombie."

"But, he is getting muscles."

"But, he's also getting a hater 'tude. Like, muscles make him better."

"Better than who? ...Or would that be whom?"

"Than anybody without them."

"I got muscles," said Tommy, flexing a chub-padded arm. "They just don't show."

"I noticed that," said Brandon. "When you jumped on me. ...You think Troy looks cool?"

Tommy shrugged. "If you like muscles that show, I guess. But, looking cool and being cool don't always come in the same

47

package."

"I've noticed that, too," agreed Brandon. "...So, how come you've never been shy? Like, you never wear a shirt."

"Maybe 'cause you never dissed me in my formative years."

"Couldn't have just been that."

Tommy smiled. "You were the first friend I ever had. And always the best. ...I have to kill you now."

"So, you think being fat is cool?"

"You just said I was... and bitchin' and boss."

"I didn't mean *because* you're fat, I mean because you're you."

"If I wasn't fat I'd be somebody else. Like, if you had muscles you might be Troy."

Brandon spread his arms and puffed his chest. "Hey, I have muscles!"

Tommy patted Brandon's chest as if to humor him. "Yeah, but your brain is what's really ripped."

"Think Troy's a hater?" asked Brandon, deflating.

"I think he's been taking hater lessons ever since he got them weights."

"Those weights."

"Dumb-bells, and they're working."

"Guess you know a lot about fat."

"More than a Master's, less than a Ph.D." Tommy stretched out beside Brandon and pillowed his head on his arms. "So, what's it like in your school?"

"Public school is one-size-fits-all, like cheap clothes that don't fit anyone. And now I'm one of the smallest dudes instead of one of the biggest."

"Da Beast not have dat problem yet. ...Get your writing class?"

"Yeah, and it's totally boss. Makes up for all the mookie shit."

"You gonna take a swim?" asked Tommy. "I'm just about done with the lawn."

"How much Da Beast charge for mowing Bucky's?"

"Five and a beer."

"Deal." Brandon got up and brushed back his hair. "I'll be in the pool."

48

Tommy climbed back on the tractor and plugged the buds in his ears. "For you, *señor,* I will mow like the wind."

SEVEN

The drapes were drawn to keep out the sun, and the huge living room was a chamber of shadows as Brandon came in and took off his pack. He dropped it on the coffee table atop the latest magazines -- *Smithsonian, National Geographic, Computing, People*, and *Mother Jones* -- that no one actually read. The air-conditioner murmured low while Tommy's tractor droned outside grazing Brandon's grass. Brandon walked down a long hallway, past his father's dim-lit den and four enormous bedrooms, into the spacious ranch-style kitchen. There was a massive double-door fridge, a mighty dishwasher, a vast island range, a big microwave, a four-slice toaster, plus various blenders and other machines, many still mysteries to Brandon because his mom never used them.

Sunlight sparkled the swimming pool and shimmered in through sliding glass doors that opened onto the patio. It winked on rows of bright copper pans that hung from racks above the range, and frolicked in ripples around the room like being in an aquarium. Brandon opened the monster fridge to snag a bottle of San Miguel beer. He popped the cap and leaned way back to guzzle it down as fast as he could... that first icy swallow was always the best.

He felt his tummy grow heavy and round, sticking out a bit like Zach's, though nothing that extreme. His jeans slipped down to an indecent level like a little kid would wear them, a comfortable, careless, mook-it-all feeling like the 1960s phrase of letting it all hang out. He killed the bottle and sucked a breath, then stripped like a savage gone back to the wild, scattering clothes across the tiles, jeans, shorts, sneaks and socks.

50

The patio brick was hot underfoot, but that was a pleasant kind of pain, like dancing across a broiling beach to meet the cool embrace of the sea. He dove in the pool, not using the board, and swam like a dolphin escaped from a net, rolling, spinning, then diving down deep, pushing up from the bottom and rocketing skyward to burst from the water and grab the board. He did a few chin-ups hanging there, enjoying the feeling of strength in his arms, then dropped in the water to float on his back.

He wished Tommy was with him; it would have been cool to play right now, transforming themselves into Bucky and Beast, the Free Mutant Boys of Beastworld. Maybe that wasn't very mature, but Brandon was tired of being fourteen, like wearing new clothes that didn't fit, small, too tight, and restrictive.

He swam to a floating lounge chair and climbed aboard to sprawl in the sun... maybe obscenely, his shaft half erect and thrusting skyward, but who gave a mook. Lapping waves made soothing sounds while bees bumbled over the flowerbeds that lined the backyard fence, blending their hum with the droning mower and making a drowsy duet. The sky was so clear you could almost fall in, and the smell of cut grass was twice as sweet since Tommy was doing the work.

It was good to be back in a peaceful place after all the confusion and hassle today. The warm beer buzz and heat of the sun was bringing his body to throbbing life, but he could enjoy that without the effort of manual manipulation. He thought up a lot of stories like this, here on his back, adrift in the water, but most got away before he could catch them, escaping between the pool and computer like dreams often vanished when leaving your bed.

Becoming "Special" had been kind of cool, walking the track with the friendly fat boys -- Jason had thankfully lagged behind -- sharing sodas and candy bars smuggled in by little T-Rex, while the "normal" kids bashed and battered each other, goaded and spurred by the bellowing coach who might have been paid for making pain and each bloody nose was a bonus.

The concept was kind of barbaric... forcing kids to fight each other. Were sports a "healthy alternative to violence?" Or, were they really just surrogate wars where none of the wounds were supposed to be fatal and only your pride got murdered or maimed on the field of somebody else's honor?

Brandon's brother had been on a team until his Junior year, but had finally quit in disgust. What were sports all about, he'd said: if you lost, you got cursed by a sadistic goon, called a sissy, a wimp, or worse for losing to another goon's team. If you won, the *goon* got a cheap tin trophy to gather dust in his office. Sports were as old as the human race... but so were violence, hate, and wars.

Brandon supposed he could fight in a war, carry a gun and kill for a cause if there was anything worthy to win... like "freedom and justice for all." But, what did he care if victory went to the Shirts or the Skins? He wasn't afraid of getting hurt; he'd splattered gallons of skater blood on most of the sidewalks in West Santa Cruz. But, nobody *told* him to bust a move, and nobody got in his face if he failed and ordered him to do it again. And, nobody told him when to fight, or when it was smarter to run away and live to fight another day. He thought of the surfers out off the Point: sometimes they dissed and cursed each other, and he'd seen a few fights in the parking lot, but mostly it was them and the sea, and nobody told them what waves to ride, or belittled them if they didn't.

Who had invented surfing, he wondered? Hawaiians, yeah, but kids or adults? No doubt it must have been a kid who'd nailed a set of roller skate wheels onto a piece of wooden plank, and probably, promptly, fell on his ass... "busted his buns" like an ancient Beach Boys song. But had anyone yelled at him to get up? To "be a man," to do it again, to skin his knees and shred his elbows and batter himself to a bloody mess until he learned to master his plank and other kids thought it was cool.

That had been in the 1960s... Brandon had read it somewhere. Who was that kid who'd invented the skateboard and found his cool on steel wheels? Legend said he'd been a surfer who'd lost his board on hungry rocks. Some said it had happened in Santa Cruz.

Brandon thought of Bosco, a natural transition. Bosco was a star athlete, yet he didn't rate shit in the eyes of the coach. Surfing wasn't a team sport, and Bosco didn't *look* like a winner. And fat kids weren't supposed to win no matter what the game.

Troy dissed Bosco for being fat -- not to his face, of course -- yet Troy had looked like an awed little kid when Bosco had signed his magazine cover. Troy would pin it up in his room; a fat boy riding a monster wave, rolly and brown in cutoff jeans -- the coolest kind of fat to be -- a red long-board beneath his feet, a watery wall of blue at his back. But Troy couldn't accept Bosco's body.

Because it blew the health-nazi image of how a winner should look.

Lunch had been a dilemma for Troy, being seen with the blubber boys, everyone from Special Ed except for dismal Jason Gray who'd slunk away to "diet." On the other hand, being seen with Bosco was worth a hundred points of cool. But the other fat dudes were negative numbers on anybody's coolness chart.

And now maybe Brandon was, too?

He'd definitely dusted most of his cool by choosing to be Special. He might have been forgiven for that -- *too bad about Brandon, stuck with the fatties, but, hey, he hurt himself lifting weights* -- but he'd blown that option by staying with them. He'd showered down in the "Pig Pen," like bathing with a gang of Beasts in an echoing watery cave. And he'd laughed along with the fat boys, too. Like, fat kids had any right to laugh.

That was a total coolness killer.

For anyone but Bosco.

Bosco was an enigma; something you couldn't define. He was one of those dudes who could do what he wanted but nobody really knew why. He was cool for many other reasons besides because he surfed... maybe not to dudes like Troy, but other people felt it. A sort of cool attraction that couldn't be explained. But he didn't seem to care about cool, equally friendly to everyone, grinning his goofy beaver grin from under his messy mop of hair. The surfers all seemed to know who he was -- the Pacific Championship winner -- yet he didn't seem to have any friends who knew him personally.

But, whoever he was he was cool, which meant he was free to *be* who he was... whatever that was. If he wanted to hang with the fat boys -- even though he wasn't *that* fat -- nobody would hold it against him.

But, Brandon was no one, nobody knew him, and muscles and tans were a dime a dozen in sunny seaside Santa Cruz. Zach hadn't even remembered his face from the hundreds of other pseudo-surfers hanging at the beach. Bosco could blow off the fat boys tomorrow and no one would even remember, but Brandon's choice of first-day friends was bar-coded onto his forehead.

Rex was a technical loser, too, if only because of his *lack* of size. He'd stuck to Brandon like Super Glue, at Brandon's side while walk-ing the track, and shyly close while showering. He'd never been naked with other dudes, though he hadn't tried to hide his chest – or in his case the lack of one -- like dorky Jason Gray. He'd traded lockers with some other kid and moved down into the Pig Pen... the last and least desirable lockers farthest from the entrance door. Bosco and Zach had also traded, along with Carlos and Kelvin. But what could you do when you looked eleven yet had all the needs of being thirteen? Find a friend and hang on tight? Survival of the littlest?

But that was cool because Rex was cool -- at least among the fat boys -- and Brandon's cool was probably toast.

Funny, he thought, adrift in the sky, in a way it was like a relief. He'd found a place from which to observe, and still had cool com-panions. He might even be an enigma himself, a dude who'd chosen not to be chosen; a dude who hadn't wagged his tail and begged somebody to throw him a bone. A dude who'd rejected potential rejection before the rejectors rejected him.

Travis White was another enigma. Travis surprised him at every turn... or was it Brandon who went the wrong way and had to make a one-eighty? It wasn't until the last bell had rung that Brandon asked where Travis lived. By then he'd expected to be surprised... like, Travis lived in Santa Cruz Gardens or some other nice suburban site. So, it had been a surprise in reverse to find that he lived in The Flats.

Kelvin lived with Travis. Brandon hadn't asked why, though he'd heard all the usual black TV tales about fathers in prison and mothers on crack. But Kelvin had taken a different bus because of a doctor's appointment. There really was something wrong with his heart... didn't that happen to crack babies?

It had been a long day of decisions for Brandon, like wandering lost in a labyrinth where his every move was videotaped to be used against him in coolness court. His last decision had been on the bus... it was filling up fast but not yet full, and Travis spread out when he sat down, his blubber taking up most of a seat. This forced another decision on Brandon... squeezing himself beside his new friend, or taking a seat across the aisle. It should have been a simple choice, and yet it was a dilemma.

One: it would look kind of funny.

Two: it would look kind of gay.

Three: would Travis think he was gay?

Four: would Travis feel betrayed if Brandon didn't sit beside him?

And Travis wouldn't give him a clue!

He'd boarded the bus ahead of Brandon, puffing hard and pouring sweat from the effort of walking across the quad. It had taken a lot more panting and puffing to get all his fat up the bus's steps. Brandon had wanted to help, but wasn't sure what to do... try to push Travis's mammoth behind? That sure as mook wouldn't look cool. There were a lot of snickers and smirks as Travis had finally struggled aboard and waddled his way to the first empty seat. The bus had rocked and rolled a bit. Then he'd just gazed out the window, as if there was anything to see except parents in minivans picking up kids. Brandon had almost felt angry that Travis wouldn't clue him... did he even want Brandon's company on his way back to the black universe? Was he being polite because of his size, not wanting Brandon to suffer beside him? Or was it because of Brandon's color. ...Or maybe the lack of it?

Brandon had dithered like that for a minute, then jammed himself to Travis's side, like shoving into hot sweaty Jell-O. Then he'd thought he'd blown it because part of his bottom was still in the aisle, which made him look ridiculous.

But, Travis had made a little more room by squeezing himself to the bus's side and draping an arm across the seat back. Brandon got most of his butt on the seat, though it looked gay to be pressed against Travis, the dude's huge arm across his shoulders... or looking like it was. Then he had glanced across the aisle and saw the blond girl in the leather sandals who might have smiled at him that morning. She didn't seem to notice him now. Outside he saw Troy in his mother's Beamer -- naturally without a shirt -- and the girl was probably watching him. Maybe she'd given up on Brandon... since he seemed to have a boyfriend?

Travis had chuckled.

"What's funny?" Brandon had demanded, as if that didn't seem obvious.

But, Travis was looking out the window. "Check out the time machine."

Brandon had peered around Travis's chest, which took a lot of peering around. Bosco's ride had arrived; an incredibly battered Volkswagen van with a surfboard strapped to its roof. The van looked like a 60s model, and the surfboard might have been even older, a redwood monster as long as the truck and painted an impudent, raving red with a grinning, cigar-smoking rat on its nose... the board in the magazine picture.

Brandon couldn't see the van's driver, but someone handed Bosco a beer -- looked like a Budweiser long-neck -- a blatant defiance, a spit-in-your-face, of the plainly posted DRUG FREE ZONE. Bosco had lost his hoodie, and his bobby-breasted chubbiness was also a kind of defiance. The van clattered off in a cloud blue smoke, maybe another defiance.

"You believe in time travel?" Brandon had asked, as the rusty old van disappeared down the hill.

Travis had looked thoughtful. "Somebody like Bosco could make me believe. You check out his sneaks today? They're genuine U.S. Keds."

"Never heard of 'em."

"They haven't been made for centuries."

"Maybe they're reproductions? Like punks and emos wear."

"Nope," said Travis. "They're on the real. The only others I ever saw were in an antique shop. ...You check the brand on his hoodie?"

"There wasn't any," said Brandon. "At least not where you could see it. And his cutoffs were Levis 501s. No way to tell how old they were."

"Make a sweet story, huh?"

Brandon had considered. "Like... 'The Dude Who Surfed Time?' Or something like that?"

"Maybe 'The Time Surfer-boy?'"

"Yeah, that sounds better."

Travis had looked thoughtful again. "Maybe he doesn't know it's the future? That's why he's so lost in space. 'Spaced-out' is a '60s expression."

"Late sixties," said Brandon. "Kinda post-surf. The psychedelic era. 'Love, peace and stop the war'... the Vietnam war."

"I hate to say duh," said Travis.

"Like that Jimi Hendrix song about never hearing surf music again."

"You like Jimi?"

"Yeah, I have three of his albums."

"There was a TV show," said Travis. "*Lost In Space*. That was in the early sixties."

Brandon smiled. "Not many people would know that."

"I watch a lot of classic TV."

"And write?"

"Another little thing I do. And I like ghost stories."

"Yeah, me too. And fantasy. Mutants and stuff."

Travis had chuckled again. "I kinda guessed that already."

"Well..." said Brandon, "go with the flow. Like, maybe Bosco's a ghost? Like, maybe he drowned a long time ago but he always comes back for his first day of school? He had enough sand in his hair to be drowned... I saw a drowned kid on the beach last year, all covered with sand and seaweed. ...And he wasn't on the school computer. They couldn't find his schedule. And his name was *penciled* on the roll in Mr. Rosenberg's class. Like he's not on anybody's grid."

"Okay," said Travis. "But, explain the magazine cover. And winning that surfing contest in June. It's not like he doesn't exist here and now."

Brandon had thought for a moment as the bus started up and

pulled away. "Well... this was the best summer of his life. Bosco said that, remember? Or that summer was. Whenever it was. When surfers still rode long-boards... like, around 1963. Surfers dressed like him in those days, and wore their hair shaggy like his. And they drove old vans like he got in."

"Speaking of which," said Travis. "Who was driving? Another ghost?"

"Didn't you see?"

"All I saw was a hand with a beer. But it had skin on it."

"Anyway," Brandon went on, "it was such a cool summer... say, in 1963... that he keeps coming back to live it again. Being reborn like he said. Waking up on a beach."

"Okay," said Travis again. "But, you gotta respect the genre. Could a ghost from 1963 win a surfing contest today?"

"It's doable," said Brandon. "People have ridden in ghost trains. And there was the ghost of a truck driver who picked up hitchhikers at night. Ghosts can interact with the living and even seem to have substance." He'd laughed. "And Bosco has lots of that."

Travis had considered. "Doesn't seem fair to the living surfers, being beat-out by a ghost."

"Well," said Brandon. "Assuming he didn't use ghostly powers, his skills would be decades out of date. And he won it on a long-board. I don't know much about surfing, but a long-board is pretty slow and clumsy compared to what they ride today. That would be more like a handicap."

"Kinda like being fat."

"He's not *that* fat. ...Oh sorry, man."

"I'm pretty slow and clumsy, too, in case you haven't noticed."

"Not where it counts, and I have noticed that."

"Thanks."

"The plot needs some work," said Brandon. "But it's a cool idea."

"You ever collaborate?"

"We could," said Brandon. "Maybe for the semester story that Mr. Akida was talking about? The one that counts for half our grade." Brandon had thought for a moment. "Um, you don't *really* think Bosco's a ghost?"

58

Travis had chuckled again. "Guess we'll know if comes back tomorrow. ...Or maybe not."

EIGHT

Brandon opened his eyes to the infinite sky. He must have dozed off adrift in the pool, lulled by the gentle liquid sounds. For a moment he felt confused, as if he was floating face-down in the water instead of gazing up into space, suspended above an ocean abyss of fathomless crystal blue. Slowly he sorted his thoughts, recalling where his mind had been before he'd fallen asleep.

Mr. Akida had told the class that a writer had to look at life from many different perspectives, think new thoughts and meet new people, try new things and take a few chances, or what would he have to write about that hadn't been written before? And a writer had to break the rules, maybe become an outlaw – maybe even a terrorist -- who wrote as if words were powerful weapons, or else bad things would never change because no one would *know* they were wrong.

Brandon, adrift, considered that, wondering if he had what it took to be a real writer. He'd already chosen to be an outlaw by hanging with the fat boys. Could he also become a terrorist?

But, what would be his cause?

He rolled off the lounge, swam a few strokes, and climbed the steps out of the pool, then padded wetly into the kitchen, dripping a trail across the tiles, snagged another beer from the fridge and leaned way back to chug it down.

Someone grabbed him from behind!

His mind flashed to Carlos the gang boy. Had Carlos decided to take revenge for Brandon stripping him on the beach? Brandon expected a knife at his throat. A wicked switchblade, an expert slash, and his blood gushing over the floor.

60

"Do I owe you, punk?" a voice demanded.

Brandon relaxed. He'd nearly choked. An amber trickle ran down his chin to spatter his chest with golden foam. He swallowed what remained in his mouth and managed to suck a breath. "Ya think?" he gasped. "I covered your ass when you scratched the Saab. Told mom I did it, remember?"

His arms stayed pinned for another few seconds, then his attacker released him and Brandon turned to face his brother.

"That's good for *one* beer," conceded Chad Williams, seventeen and buff as a brick with high, jutting pecs and six-pack abs. He was tanned and shirtless in new Tommy jeans, showing six inches of blue boxer shorts. Basically he was a bigger Brandon, except for less hair and a lot more muscle. "But why should I take the heat for two?"

"Three," said Brandon. "And I can't back the car out anymore."

Chad inspected the fridge. "What are you talking about, dork? I see four bottles in there. You haven't been in public school long enough for your brain to rot. ...More than it already has."

"I owe Tommy one for mowing the lawn."

"*Why* is he mowing our lawn, by the way? Dad got the new Toro last month. Isn't it good enough for you? Just one cup holder?"

"'Cause I'm paying him five and a beer," said Brandon.

Chad shook his head. "They didn't let me have one beer a day until I turned sixteen. So, who the hell died and made you a prince? ...And look at the freakin' mess you made! Water all over the freakin' floor! Your freakin' clothes all over the place! And your freakin' pack on the coffee table! ...And when are you gonna cut your hair? You look like an underdeveloped girl."

Brandon took a sip of beer. "I'm cuter than your last girlfriend."

"Only in retrospect. Now get the mop and clean up your mess! ...And give me the rest of that beer! You wanna get a big fat belly?" Chad snatched the bottle and poked Brandon's tummy. "You've almost got one already! Quit slouching and suck it in, stupid! Start paying attention to how you look or nobody's gonna like you!"

"What about you?" laughed Brandon, doing neither as Chad killed the bottle.

"I work out!" retorted Chad. "You just lay around and read...

when you're not on your computer or jacking-off in your room. Or sitting on your ass and writing fantasy stories."

"So, how do I have any time to skate?" Brandon reached for another beer.

"Touch it and painfully die!" roared Chad.

"You owe me, mook-head!" Brandon yelled back. "I saw you twice at school today and I didn't embarrass you by acknowledging you're my brother, did I? And once was with a girl... who wasn't under-developed."

Chad smiled a little. "So, how did it go?"

"Brandon lives, ta-da. Didn't get in any fights."

"Don't," said Chad. "They play for keeps in jungle-land. The brown dudes have knives and the black ones have guns."

Brandon frowned. He tried not to stereotype people, yet the first thing he'd thought when grabbed from behind was a Mexican dude with a knife. "Well, the whiteys sell most of the drugs."

"Making connections already?" asked Chad.

"Oh, shut up."

Chad shrugged. "You'll learn, my mentally-challenged child. I remember my first day of high school..."

"Oh, puh-leeeeze, grampaw! Should I sit on your knee while you reminisce?"

"Should I sit on your face while I kick your ass? Mom wanted you in a private high school. ...Or don't you remember that little war? You come home all beat up, or cut up, or shot... or start getting high all the time again... and it's back to a private school, little prince, or maybe some kind of academy for over-privileged underachievers."

"I'm sure they have way better drugs," said Brandon.

"I'm sure you would know."

Brandon snagged another bottle. "So, how come you're in public school?"

"'Cause I made the same mistake you're making. I wanted to be with my 'normal friends.' Like some clueless kid on a TV show... gets a chance at a decent school but wants to be a 'regular guy,' so he throws away a good education for a few wasted years with the Proles. Like, those kind of friends really matter. Like, they're gonna be useful in life."

"Like the kind of friends you have?"

"Friends aren't forever."

"Real ones are."

"Only in stories," said Chad. "And how would you know about forever? You're only stupid fourteen." Then he shrugged. "I blew it, man, but you don't have to."

"But you get better grades than I ever did."

"Oh, that really counts with college admissions, getting A's in a suckhole school where they graduate goons who can't even read their ass-wipe diplomas."

"But you're going to Stanford next year."

"'Cause mom and dad have money, moron. But I'm still gonna start with a strike against me for going to Trailer-Trash High." Chad shook his head. "Maybe you'll get a clue this year about how life really works. And getting beat up a few times might help. Just don't expect me to do any paybacks."

"Um, did you?" asked Brandon."

"Get beat up? Ya think, Goldilocks."

"How come you never said anything?"

"It's not like a medal of honor. Besides, I didn't want mom to know. For reasons already mentioned. Why do you think I got my weights?"

"I thought you buffed-up to get girls."

"It helps with that, too... as you apparently noticed today. But mass is like a defense in school."

Tommy came bobbling in. "The lawn is done."

"The lawn is finished," said Brandon.

"The lawn is completed," said Tommy.

Brandon gave him the bottle. "Thanks, man."

"Hey," growled Chad. "Go on a diet, blubber-boy! Before your belly hangs down to your knees!"

"I'm on one now," Tommy replied, popping the cap and gulping beer.

"You're obese!"

"Nah, I'm just fat. ...Can I take a swim, Brandon?"

"Since when do you have to ask?"

Chad shook his head. "Don't you have a pool of your own? Or can't you manage to walk that far lugging all your lard?"

"So carry me home, *Jerk*-you-lees."

"You can't even keep your jeans on your ass!"

"Look who's talking, sagger-boy!"

"With me it's a choice, for you it's a life."

"Try getting a life," said Tommy. "And these jeans are coming off my ass, so close your eyes if it bothers you, mook. Size does matter."

"Excuse me?" said Chad. "Have I just been mooked by a fat little kid who can't even see his own dick?"

"Felt my lips move when I mooked ya, mook. And I don't need to see it to put it to use in all the ways nature intended... or at least, like your frustrated self, most of them so far."

"...How would...?" Chad's cheeks reddened a bit. "If I had an ass as big as yours I wouldn't be showing it off!"

"You're showing off all you got right now, which isn't a pretty sight, and I wasn't talking about my ass."

"Oh, gimmie a break you're only twelve!"

"So, what's your excuse, little man?"

Chad paused, maybe counting to ten. "Don't piss in my pool, blubber-boy. And buy yourself a bra!"

Tommy aggressively thrust out his breasts. "You know you want these desperately 'cause you never touched anything like 'em before except in your hydraulic dreams."

"I know I want 'em out of here along with all the rest of your fat!"

"Remember that when you're thirty," said Tommy, "and regretting what you didn't do when the time was right."

"Out!" Chad watched as Tommy waddled away, then gave Brandon a smirk. "Isn't he a bit young for you, even with all his development?"

"Oh, bite me, Chad."

"Seriously, you're in high school now. You shouldn't be hanging with fat little kids."

"What's being fat got to do with anything?"

"It's another strike against him. Which means it's a strike against you. You have to think of your image."

Brandon recalled the choices he'd made. "Let somebody else think about it. It's their problem, not mine."

"Oh they will," said Chad. "And they'll make it your problem if you don't look like they want you to look. You wanted to go there, you better learn that. If you don't, you die. Figuratively, or maybe for real."

"You're metaphorically-challenged," said Brandon. "But I don't think you're little."

"You think I care what a twelve-year-old says?"

"Looked like you did for a second. But, fully extended you're a bit above average according to what I've read."

"Like I needed that from you."

"You still have wet dreams?"

"Depends on who's hostessing them. ...You'd have better teachers in private school. Especially for writing."

Brandon laughed. "My teacher last year wasn't published. Didn't want to 'rush into print.' Mr. Akida has seven books out."

"Asians are smart."

"Try African, man."

"...Oh," said Chad. "So, how come he's teaching at Suckhole Central?"

"'Cause a lot of good writers aren't rich."

"Then what's the point of writing? ...Snag me a beer, pretty boy."

"You like your boys underdeveloped? And how are we gonna cover four?"

"The 'we' was noted," said Chad. "The other remark is beneath contempt. I'll score a new sixer before they get home. I know the dude at Beer Botique."

"Sounds like a useful friend."

"For this time and place."

"That's bitchin'," said Brandon. "They have five-hundred brands. I wanna check 'em all this year."

"You'll really get a big fat belly."

"Thought I had one already? There's worse things than being fat."

"Such as?"

65

"Being a stupid hater, for one. ...Or, how about fish full of mercury? Or global-warming? Or pollution? Or 'wars on terror' that are really for oil?"

"You may have a point," said Chad. "But you gotta come up with the cash for brew. And seventy-five a week isn't much. Not when you're in high school. I'm trying to live on a hundred, and I don't even smoke."

"I don't either anymore, so give that topic a funeral."

"You used to be so mookin' cute when you stumbled around in a daze all the time. ...You know smoking weed can delay puberty? Or keep you in it longer?"

"I pubered a long time ago, and it's been a delightful experience."

"You better ask dad for a raise tonight. His stock went up so it's a good time. Try for a hundred, but don't include your bus pass and lunch money. And definitely not your clothing expenses... you are a growing boy. You can still beg extra for movies and unforeseen contingencies."

Brandon handed a bottle to Chad. "You're boss, big-dog."

"Way too... boss... for a loser like you. And thanks for not knowing me today."

"Was that Lisa?" asked Brandon. "She's pretty, besides being well-developed."

"Yeah. Thanks."

"Are they real?"

"So far that's my working assumption." Chad opened the door to the three-car garage. "Just don't be drunk at dinner, okay? You laugh at dad's jokes and then he tells more. That's worse than when you were stoned all the time. Then you only smiled. ...Put the bottles in the recycle bin. ...And get this freakin' mess cleaned up."

Brandon followed his brother into the garage, empty except for a black Trans-Am, a '75 and partly restored. He studied a dusty surfboard that lay on the rafters above, its leash hanging down like a noose. "You ever gonna use that again?"

Chad got in his car. "I should sell it. I wanted to have a garage sale and get rid of all my old kid-crap, but mom won't let me. 'It's too middle-class for this neighborhood.'"

"We're upper-class?" asked Brandon.

"I've never been sure what we are. But this house is worth at least two mil with the ocean right across the street."

"So, we're millionaires?"

"Not in disposable income. We'd have to liquidate our assets... sell the house... then where would we live?"

"But we'd have all that money."

"A million or two doesn't buy much these days."

"So, what happened with surfing, Chad?"

Chad glanced up at the board. "That surfing thing is like a phase. A lot of kids go through it." He took a cigar off the car's dashboard.

"What's that?" asked Brandon.

"A cigar, boy-genius."

"What kind, mook-head?"

"Genuine Cuban. A friend of mine gets 'em cheap, and I don't ask from where."

"Another useful friend?"

"The key word is useful, remember that."

"Can I have one?"

"A useful friend? That would be a first for you."

"That's so lame it needs a crutch."

"Got ten bucks?" Chad lit the cigar with a Bic.

"Thought you said your friend got 'em cheap?"

"Retail is fifty. ...Oh, here, dork." Chad took another cigar off the dash. "The first one's always free... as you know."

"Thanks," said Brandon, taking a puff after Chad fired his lighter. "Hey, this rocks! ...So, you don't think Troy's gonna last at surfing? Like it's a phase for him?"

Chad blew smoke. "Real surfing is like a religion."

"Like, pray for surf?"

"They used to say that in the 1960s. Wait until Indian Summer's gone and the weather starts getting cold. That's when you know who's a surfer for real."

Brandon blew a smoke ring. "These are boss."

Chad cocked his head. "Where have I heard that word before?"

67

Brandon shrugged. "I heard it at school today. Must be fresh."

"Or just Fresh-man."

Brandon took another puff. "I guess you could be right about Troy. He's more into weights than surfing now. Weights and being... retch... 'healthy.' Almost like an obsession."

"Sometimes a cigar is just a cigar."

"And sometimes it isn't," said Brandon. "That's all he wants to do anymore. It's getting so mookin' boring with him. I always gotta look at his body, tell him how big his muscles are getting, feel his stupid 'ceps and pecs."

"That paints a rather gay picture," said Chad.

"I don't even think I'd care if he was. He's just getting zombie-boring."

"I know what you mean," said Chad. "I've met a few dudes who got hooked on their bodies and fell in love with themselves." Chad laughed. "Like jacking-off while flexing in a mirror."

Brandon laughed, too. "Yeah, he does. ...Think it's a phase?"

"Sometimes, I guess. But it can backfire. I've seen a few of my friends' older brothers who spent all their teen years buffing up. They stop working out after high school and all that muscle turns to fat. Like, it's better not to get too ripped or you're chained to that look for the rest of your life... at least if you want to keep your friends."

"They weren't really friends if they stopped liking you just because you got fat," said Brandon.

"Like I said, little one, you don't how the world works yet... including how shallow most people are."

"How come you never got like that? Wanted to get hella ripped?"

"I told you, it's a survival thing in my present time and place. The look gets girls and pleases the Proles... advice you should take to heart, brother dear."

"But, it isn't really you?"

"Does anybody really know who they are?"

"The answer is 42. ...Were you good at surfing?"

"Not good enough for Steamer Lane. I graduated from Capitola proficient enough for Pleasure Point... assuming Night Fighter approval... but that's not a useful accomplishment."

"So, what do you want for the board?"

Chad sighed. "Sometimes I think dad's right about kids always making the same old mistakes in every new generation. Like re-inventing the wheel every decade."

"What's wrong with that?" asked Brandon. "Experience is the best teacher, you kinda just said that yourself."

"But, learning through experience wastes a lot of your time. ...Time is important, Brandon. It's also an unforgiving bitch, but you're still too young to know it."

"Zot?"

"Four years seems like forever, huh?"

"What do you mean?"

"Until you graduate."

"...Kinda," said Brandon.

"It was for me, too. But wait till you're looking back on three. Then you'll understand. Time is like money, Brandon, don't waste it in the present on things that won't buy you a future."

"Like learning to surf?"

"Ask yourself what it gets you... learning to surf, making friends, or anything else you do in the present. Invest your present time in the future. You're not a kid anymore. Don't waste your time learning more kid-stuff because that's all in the past." Chad tossed his bottle into the glass bin. "Take the board if you want it. If you practice getting up in the pool you won't look like a total geek if you ever really go out in the ocean."

"Thanks, Chad. ...What's a Tola-Rat?"

"A cross between an elephant and a rhinoceros."

"Seriously. Is it a gang?"

"If it is, then stay away from it! ...What did you do today, anyhow? See how many thugs you could meet?"

"'Course not. I hooked with some really cool dudes. One of them is black, and another one has this bitchin' tattoo of a Tola-Rat."

"You're such an innocent babe," sighed Chad. "You hooked with a black kid and a punk with a tat! It's illegal in California. You can't get a tat until you're eighteen."

69

"He got it when he was eight."

"How charmingly trailer-trashy."

"He's not trailer-trash! And you don't even know him!"

"I know more than I want to already. You've really lived a sheltered life."

"Oh, kiss my ass!"

"Looks too much like your face. ...What's wrong with the black kid? Besides being one."

"Nothing's wrong with him, dammit! He's in my Creative Writing class. He's even got a computer. ...Are you prejudiced or something?"

"Sorry to shock you, wide-eyed-one, but I am in a practical sense."

"...Why? Mom and dad aren't. They were against Apartheid. And they wanted to keep Affirmative Action."

"That's idealism, I'm talking reality."

"The mook *are* you talking about?"

"When did they ever have black people over? Like, to dinner or parties?"

"...Guess mom and dad don't know any."

"Probably aren't any where they work. Which proves my point."

"What point?"

"About making useful friends." Chad flicked ashes from his cigar. "Life isn't a smarmy TV show where well-off kids go to suckhole schools so they can have 'regular pals.'"

"You said that already."

Chad studied his brother. "Come here, man." He got out of the car and took Brandon's shoulders. "It's like I'm seeing you three months later. You're taller now. Put on some weight... and not just your belly. You have an actual chest. And your eyes aren't even red." He shook Brandon gently. "You're okay, twink. ...Clueless and girly, but still okay." He drew Brandon against his chest for a moment. "And I love you, brother mine, even if I don't like you much."

Brandon smiled. "You can kill me now."

"Listen, kid, it's quality time. You don't know it yet, but this was the summer that changed everything."

"Zot?"

"I didn't know it either when I was your age. Not till a long time after. ...It's like a story you read to me once, about a ghost in a haunted house. But people don't know it's a ghost when they see it. Not till a long time after. It's not a ghost that haunts their present, but it haunts their future because it was part of their past."

"That's deep," said Brandon.

"I'll sue if you plagiarize it." Chad got back in the car. "Watch your back at school, pretty-boy... figuratively and literally. Don't be alone in the locker room. And be careful who you hook with. You lie down with dogs, you wake up with fleas. ...That's not being a racist, it's just a practical fact of life."

Chad shut the door. "*You're* not thinking of getting a tat? Mom had a cow when you pierced your ear! She'd have a whole litter if you got a tat!"

"That would be a herd," said Brandon. "Just wondered what Tola-Rat means."

"Probably trouble. Why didn't you ask?"

"I didn't think it would be cool."

Chad shook his head again. "You have a *lot* to learn about life. You'll probably get raped if you don't cut that hair. ...Oh, and by the way, if you're gonna sleep on the lounge in the pool, either turn on your belly or put on some shorts. This has been a message from mom."

"Zot?"

"Fully extended you're a bit above average according to what I've read."

"...Oh. ...But, that's totally normal."

"Lots of things are totally normal, but lots of people don't want to see 'em."

Brandon smiled. "Remember the Free Beach, Chad? I was eleven the last time we went."

"Yeah, and I was your age."

"Wonder how come we stopped going?"

Chad thumbed the garage door remote. "Mom and dad are getting old, but you probably haven't noticed yet."

The Trans-Am's engine fired with a roar, filling the air with eye-

71

searing smoke as the door began to rumble open. Chad clamped the cigar between his teeth and slapped the stick into reverse. "Get your ass out before the door opens and somebody sees you naked. The neighbors might think you're gay. That's all I need, a gay little brother! I'd rather have a fat one!"

NINE

C had backed out and blasted away, burning rubber, spewing smoke, and otherwise pissing the neighbors. Brandon watched the car rocket past Lighthouse Point while the door came rumbling slowly down, then he returned to the kitchen, snagged the last two beers in the fridge and buried the cardboard out of sight in the paper recycling bin.

Tommy was sprawled on the floating lounge, glistening brown in the golden sun, his head pillowed comfortably on his arms while his beer bottle stood in the water-filled pond surrounding the cave of his navel... sort of a natural cup holder.

"Hey, Tommy!" called Brandon from the kitchen doorway. "Want another beer? And there's half a jumbo pizza left."

"Mook yeah!" Tommy killed his brew with a monster gulp and tumbled into the water. He swam to the ladder and clambered out like a rolly-poly sea lion pup. "Who died and left you beer?"

"We survived our first days in strange new worlds. Bucky and Beast deserve a reward."

"What's that?" asked Tommy, pointing to Brandon's cigar.

"Besides the obvious, a genuine Cuban. Have a hit, man."

"Bitchin'," said Tommy, blowing smoke. "But I thought these were illegal?"

"Guess that makes us outlaws."

"We're terrorists on Beastworld."

"They cost fifty dollars retail."

"Guess I better inhale."

"We can save it for later." Brandon picked up his clothes from the tiles while Tommy got the mop.

73

"Beast do floor," said Tommy. "Bucky get pack off coffee table."

A few minutes later in Brandon's room, Tommy was at the computer, back in his cutoffs as much as could be, his big bubble-bottom bare in the chair, and chomping a cheesy pizza slice while speedily surfing the web. Brandon lay on his king-size bed, also back in jeans, sipping beer and reading his journal... mostly the notes he'd made about Travis. The drapes were drawn and the light was soft, a peaceful, golden, hazy glow like many summer afternoons when he'd wasted a lot of time like this back in his eighth-grade stoner days, lying here in his dim-lit room dreaming up stories he never wrote. That was a major danger of dope, it gave you lots of inspiration but seldom any inclination; peaceful submission with little ambition.

The room was large with lots of free space despite its perpetual sloppiness. The shelving system was sagging with things... books, CDs, and model cars, a game system, a massive TV. There was also a stereo and a few old toys from Brandon's past... Ninja Turtles, a Barney doll, and all the Transformer figures. The walls were adorned with posters; various rock groups, some of them classic -- one from the Fillmore his mother had stolen back in her anti-establishment days -- an auto-graphed glossy of Freddie Kruger, *Dragonball Z*, some *Elfquest* stuff, and a big surf picture called *Endless Summer* that Chad had thrown away last year.

"I wish it was endless," sighed Brandon, gazing up at the surfing scene. "This summer was over way too soon."

"They get shorter when you get older," said Tommy, his chubby fingers clattering keys with a sound like soft machine-gun fire.

"I'm starting to notice that," said Brandon. "How many hits on our site today?"

"Almost three-hundred, and most of them stayed over fifteen minutes, which means they can actually read. We're gonna need more bandwidth soon. ...Six porno spams in your mailbox. Seven more assorted shit... like, 'Lose That Ugly Fat'... so, who decides what's ugly? And, 'New Drug Lets You Eat Anything And Never Gain An Ounce'... maybe it makes you shit all the time? And, 'Do Your Friends Laugh When You Take Off Your Shirt?'... not if they're really your friends. Here's, 'Exercise In A Bottle'... like a genie pops out and magics you skinny. And of course we have 'Miracle Weight-loss Pills'... which *would* be a miracle if they worked. ...And a message from somebody called T-Rex."

"That's cool," said Brandon.

"Who's T-Rex... besides the 1970s band?"

"Another dude I met at school. I'll read it later; trash the spam."

"Not much to read, he just says you're cool and he'll see you tomorrow. ...Is he gay?"

"I don't think so, but I don't think I'd care as long he didn't want to go steady."

"That's one of the reasons you're cool." said Tommy. "Toilet time for diets and porn. Can't tell the difference anyway. ...Is he fat, too?"

"Rex? Nah. Looks like Suntop in *Elfquest*, but without the tan. He's kinda small for his age."

"Hence the name T-Rex," said Tommy. "Antithetical humor. Want me to check our guest book?"

"Nah. Don't feel like reading that stuff right now."

"Not even from girls?"

"They can wait, I sure have."

Tommy poised at the keyboard like a starship pilot preparing to warp. "Where you wanna go today? How about The Planet Of Porn? Or, Return To The Planet Of Porn? Or, Beneath The..."

"Nah," said Brandon. "It's kinda boring."

"Since when did jacking-off get boring?"

"I'm just not in the mood right now."

"Not even for Bimbos Hot 4-U?"

"They're only hot for my Visa card number."

"Any cool girls at school?" asked Tommy.

"I thought one girl was checking me out, but I might have scared her away on the bus."

"Did you try to sit beside her?"

Brandon remembered the scene on the bus, squeezing himself against Travis. "If I told you I'd have to kill you."

"That dorky, huh?"

"I think I saw her somewhere before. Maybe down at the Boardwalk."

"Stats?" asked Tommy.

"Could be a Sophomore. Maybe fifteen. Tan and blond but not a Barbie."

"Full-figured?" asked Tommy.

"I'm not sure what that means."

"Like 'husky' when people are being nice and don't wanna call a kid fat."

"Yeah," said Brandon. "Like charmingly chubby."

"A puppy tummy? I love puppy tummies!"

"Yeah," said Brandon. "But she looks like she's got a brain in her head. Like, she's thinking about something besides losing weight. ...Faded jeans, white T-shirt..."

"Tight T-shirt?"

"Tight enough," said Brandon, "without being slutty about it. And big leather sandals with tire treads."

"I seen a girl with them somewhere."

"You saw a girl with them somewhere."

"I observed a girl with them somewhere. And a puppy tummy. ...Breasts?"

"Oh yeah! And bigger than yours."

"Hey!" said Tommy.

"Just trying to paint you a picture with words."

"Use more exciting colors." Tommy jiggled his chest. "I can picture my breasts any time. Better yet I can fondle 'em and be my own fantasy. See?"

"Troy does the same thing with his pumped-up pecs."

"Different strokes, no pun intended."

Brandon watched for a moment, though the sight wasn't anything new -- Tommy was always feeling himself, jiggling, patting, stroking his fat -- and yet it sparked a new interest. "Do they feel anything like girl breasts?"

"I mookin' hope so," said Tommy, still caressing his spheres as if petting a pair of plump Tribbles. "Where did she get off the bus?"

"Beans!"

"Beans?" asked Tommy. "Sounds like a *Leave It To Beaver* synonym for shit."

Brandon shrugged. "A dude I met at school said it. But I didn't see where the girl got off; I was talking to another dude about writing a ghost story."

"Pay more attention tomorrow," said Tommy. "Pretty girls don't last forever like ghosts."

"How about girls at your school?"

"I have bigger breasts than most of 'em. But there was a hella cool eighth-grader... real chubby and *perfect* breasts! And a lot bigger than mine. And sometimes her tummy peeked out of her shirt. That always gets me hot! She smiled at me at lunch, and obviously wasn't watching her weight. This might be the year of Da Beast. I bought a pack of Trojans today. Gave one a test drive when I got home."

"You like fat girls?" asked Brandon.

"I like any girl if she talks to me nice." Tommy ate the rest of his pizza, gulped from his bottle and burped. "Three slices left."

Brandon patted his tummy. "I had that big lunch at school. And we'll probably order out tonight. Mom's been working a copyright case so she's probably too tired to cook."

"Force yourself, Bucky. Even Da Beast can't eat three. And they won't survive getting nuked again."

"Pass one over. ...Wanna have dinner with me?"

Tommy scowled. "My mom called your mom yesterday. She say no feed Da Beast no more. This mookin' diet is serious beans."

"I'll order a lot and we'll eat in here. What do you want?"

"So much food and so little time. ...Lamb chops with mint sauce. Ranch on a jumbo chef salad. Mashed potatoes and gravy. Corn on the cob. Zucchini, green beans, and... just call me weird... that buttered broccoli casserole."

"Weird. How about dessert?"

"You want me to keep getting fatter?"

"...Oh, sorry."

"Hey, I'm kidding. ...Ben and Jerrys. Cherries Garcia... um, no, the strawberry shortcake. ...Better yet, get both."

"Do *you* want to keep getting fatter?"

"I'm not a gainer; for me fat just happens. But I do happen to like it."

77

Brandon cocked his head. "What's a gainer?"

"Somebody who wants to get fat and/or fatter."

"But, you like being fat. And you gained twenty more pounds this summer."

"But I didn't get fatter on purpose."

Brandon keyed an invisible microphone. "Bucky to Beast: I'm a little off-course. Talk me in for a landing. Over."

Tommy spoke into the mouse. "Beast to Bucky: a gainer is someone who wants to get fat. And/or fatter. Over."

"Why would somebody want to get fat? And/or fatter, over? ...Not that there's anything wrong with it."

"Was the latter to spare my feelings? Over."

"Affirmative. Over."

Tommy put down the mouse. "'Cause they like being fat." He held up a hand. "I already know what you're gonna say about when I stuffed myself all the time. But then I was just a little kid who was trying to fight his mommy."

"Fight your mom?" asked Brandon.

"Yeah," said Tommy. "I was fighting back at her the only way I could."

"'Cause you wanted to be fat?"

"No... and listen carefully... 'cause I wanted to be *me*. But me wasn't good enough for her. Like something she ordered off the web that didn't come in the size she wanted, but she couldn't send it back, so she tried to make me fit. ...Hey, I made a pun."

Brandon finished his pizza slice. "That sounds mean. Your mom's not mean."

"When you're little it's mean," said Tommy. "Every time she'd say, 'pull down your shirt, your tummy's showing,' she was telling me to hide myself 'cause I didn't fit her mental model of how a kid should look. My body... me... was embarrassing her. Like, wearing a shirt saying I'm with stupid. So she kept trying to make me fit and it turned into a war. And I've been fighting it since I was five."

Brandon picked up his journal and scribbled *wars on kids to make them fit*. "That could mook up a childhood."

"It's mookin' up a lot of them. But that's not really gaining," said

Tommy. "Though it might trigger gaining. But, real gaining usually starts when a kid is a little older."

Brandon poised his pen. "Age has something to do with gaining?"

"There's lots of grownup gainers, but most gainers start in their early teens, or a little younger. Or at least start wanting to."

"Like, in puberty?"

"I hate that word for some reason."

"Yeah," said Brandon, making more notes. "Adults overuse it to explain anything they don't understand about kids. Like, 'going through a phase.'"

"You helped me get through it," said Tommy.

"Really?"

Tommy laughed. "Mom's no good with boy-stuff. Just say erection and she drops a dish. Sometimes I wonder how I was conceived."

"Glad I could help with the puberty thing."

"Glad you were there. And thanks for all the jacking-off lessons."

"Thought you learned that off the Internet like everybody else."

"Did you?"

"Fortunately I have a big brother who mastered in masturbation."

"Some things are learned better with personal trainers. ...But this new diet isn't gonna work any more than the others did. Most diets don't, 'specially on kids. They just gain back their old weight after their parents stop starving 'em, and usually gain even more. It's the body's defense against famine. That's what my last doctor told my mom. He said I was 'clinically obese,' but there wasn't a mookin' thing wrong with me."

"What did she do?"

"Got a new doctor. She always does if they say I'm okay. Like, she *wants* 'em to say I'm not healthy so she can keep trying to make me lose weight. Which means I keep getting fatter. In clinical terms that's a syndrome."

"But you said it was little-kid stuff."

"It's like when you're too old to spank anymore but your 'rents haven't figured that out." Tommy picked up a pizza slice. "So, I'm gonna have to get even fatter to make her stop trying to make me skinny."

"But doesn't that make you a gainer?" asked Brandon. "Now that you're older and know what you're doing?"

"Nah, 'cause I'm not getting fatter for me."

"Beast, I'm really lost in space."

Tommy looked thoughtful. "What happened today anyhow? Did you suddenly wake up and notice fat kids?" He laughed. "We're having an 'obesity epidemic,' which is a stupid thing to say 'cause being fat is not a disease you catch from somebody else."

"I told that to Troy today," said Brandon. "But they make it sound like an epidemic and something that needs to be cured. About every other TV commercial is a diet plan or a weight-loss pill."

"There's an epidemic of brainwashing people to make 'em obsess about getting skinny and hating anybody who's not."

"Hate is viral," said Brandon. "And maybe the oldest disease in the world."

"And it's killed a lot more people than any disease."

Brandon scribbled more notes. "But isn't over-eating like a substitute for something?"

"For good friends, good parents, good pastimes, good sex?"

"Slow down," said Brandon, still writing. "So, what are you missing?"

"The sex could be better... or so I've been told. I think I've done everything with myself..." He smiled, "and with you, any normal straight dude could do, and I'm not into rubber or farm animals."

Brandon scanned what he'd written. "Okay: people are being brainwashed to make kids look like they're told they should look and hate anybody who isn't or won't... but I still don't understand gaining."

"Beast will now educate Bucky." Tommy flexed his fingers and poised them over the keyboard. "Rocketing into a fat universe." Then he paused. "Brandon?"

"Yeah?"

"How come you never dissed me?"

"For what?"

"For duh."

"There wasn't anything to dis. You're cool, smart, and fun to be with. ...I have to kill you now."

"At least I'll die fulfilled... there's a word I like."

"I guess it works both ways," said Brandon. "Like, what you said when I first got home... because I never dissed you, you didn't think there was anything to dis."

"Yeah, but mom did," said Tommy. "But she didn't count 'cause I didn't trust her. She wasn't trying to make me 'healthy,' she was only trying to make me skinny so haters wouldn't hate on *her*. But right next door was this boss dude, Brandon, who liked Tommy for who he was. ...You can kill me now."

"Then I wouldn't have a bitchin' friend."

"Thanks," said Tommy. "It's like fat acceptance."

"Zot?"

"You're not prejudiced against fat people, and don't believe you're supposed to be no matter what society says."

Brandon recalled the events of the day and the friends he'd made at school. "But you were the only fat friend I had. And sometimes my only friend. Like, when I was staying high all the time and Troy stopped coming over."

Tommy shrugged. "You were still you, just not all there. Like part of you in another dimension but still enough in this one to like."

"Thanks. And you were always my best friend. ...I really have to kill you now."

"Wanna talk some more about fat first?"

"Guess it's one of your favorite subjects."

"Ironically," said Tommy, "It didn't used to be. I didn't think much about being fat, except when mom dissed me, or some hater did."

"But you said that happens a lot."

"Only in the last few years. For a while I thought it was 'cause I was older... going more places and doing more stuff. But it seems like I'm meeting my mom everywhere, only most of 'em aren't as nice." Tommy fingered the mouse. "Guess you never seen fat-acceptance sites? Except for ours."

"You mean sites with fat and chubby girls? I've been to a few.

81

They're kinda... well, huggable."

"You shoulda seen this eighth-grader today!"

"But, what did you mean, 'except ours?'"

"Don't you ever read our guest book?"

"What's that got to do with fat?"

Tommy tapped keys to call up the home page of Bucky and Beast, a graphic adventure. Tommy did the layout and Brandon wrote the stories. They'd taken selfies of themselves at Natural Bridges Beach, a place with lofty sandstone cliffs and strangely-shaped formations. Both wore cutoffs and carried spears, and their long hair gave them a young warrior look, especially when the wind was blowing. The beach re-sembled an alien planet, and Tommy had tweaked the colors, tinting the sky a lavender shade and adding a second sun. The opening scene showed Bucky and Beast poised on a cliff overlooking the sea.

Brandon came over to look at the screen. Tommy pointed. "How many fat kids have you seen like me having cool adventures? And without a shirt?"

"Never saw any as cool as you. ...I really, really have to kill you."

"Well," said Tommy. "The fat kids you see on TV or in movies are mostly the hero's dorky friends. Or maybe a loyal sidekick at best."

"Like Bucky *and* Beast?"

"It looks better on the marquee. But name me a TV show or movie that doesn't at least make fat kids look dorky."

"What about *Heavyweights?*"

"Full of stereotypes," said Tommy. "Same with Chunk in *The Goonies*... likeable but dorky. And he wasn't *that* fat."

"...Well, there's Mikey in *Recess*. He's really cool. And there's Fat Albert."

"But, they still show 'em eating a lot."

"You eat a lot."

"Sure," said Tommy. "But I wouldn't stop to have a burger if you were about to get vaporized. And *why* does a fat kid eating always get the laugh-track? Like Larry Mondello in *Leave It To Beaver*. Like, put a cheeseburger in your hand and nobody even smiles. But, just put a jelly bean in mine and people are wetting themselves."

82

"I never thought of that," said Brandon.

"Anyway..." Tommy opened the guest book. "Check this out: 'Phattest site on the web, dudes!' ...And here's another one: 'Hi, Beast, I'm eleven and almost as fat as you. You look wicked cool. Since I found your site I have been going to the beach and losing my shirt."

"What about this one?" asked Brandon. "'Buy a bra, fatso!'"

Tommy shrugged. "Ever notice that? If you coughed up some ancient hairball, like calling somebody a skeezer, *you'd* be the one who'd look like a geek. But, calling a fat kid fatso, or making bra jokes is cool to haters, even though it's been said a billion times."

"What's wrong with skeezer?" asked Brandon. "I just heard it today."

"My dad used to say that sometimes, so I figured it's gotta be Stone Age."

"Maybe it's coming back?" said Brandon. "But the same thing goes for words like nigger. That's gotta be the oldest hate-speak, but stupid haters still say it." He took the mouse and scrolled the screen. "Most of those posts are from little kids. ...'I'm eight, I'm ten, I'm seven.'"

"'I'm fifteen,'" said Tommy, pointing to another post. "And here's one who's thirteen, and one who's fourteen."

"What's your point?" asked Brandon.

"Except for a few stupid haters, those kids all like what we're doing... which is building a fat-acceptance site."

"Hey," said Brandon. "Have I been used?"

"Zot?"

"I thought we built our site 'cause it's cool? Not to make fat kids feel good."

"We *did* build our site 'cause it's cool," said Tommy. "But, what's wrong with giving fat kids a hero?" He thumbed his chest. "Such as yours truly?"

"...Nothing," said Brandon. "But it's like you had a secret agenda. You could have told me about this stuff so I could have helped... written more fat stuff into the story."

"No offense, Brandon, but you don't know anything about being fat. Isn't one of the rules of good writing to only write about what you know?"

"That's one of the bad rules of writing," said Brandon. "The good rule is, if you don't know, don't guess. Do your research and get your facts right."

"That's still my point," said Tommy. "Not only are you not fat, but you never did any research, so how could you write about being fat with any degree of veracity?"

"How about this for a start?" Brandon cupped one of Tommy's breasts. "Damn, no wonder you like 'em!"

"They come as a set, y'know?" said Tommy. "We don't want the other one to get jealous."

Brandon captured the other orb, which felt like holding a warm balloon softly inflated with Jell-O. Of course he'd touched them countless times in the course of everyday contact with Tommy, including wrestling and play, but despite trying to be objective now found himself becoming aroused. He felt his cheeks flush, yet didn't want to release what he held.

Tommy smiled. "That feels hot to me, too. Wish you'd done it a long time ago?"

Brandon finally forced himself to relinquish what part of him wanted to cherish. "Wouldn't you have thought I was weird?"

"I kinda thought it was weird you didn't. Lots of dudes want to cop a feel."

"Guess I got used to seeing 'em. ...Besides, you're like my little brother."

"I'm not little anymore." Tommy stood up. "Now give me a big brother hug."

Feeling strangely shy, Brandon put his arms around Tommy and drew the boy against him. He supposed it was an experiment, but again found he wasn't staying detached, though the adjectives that came to mind were:

"Soft, warm... and friendly," he murmured.

"Close your eyes," said Tommy. "And free-associate."

Instead, Brandon let go and stepped back. "That might not be safe."

"For who? ...Or would that be whom?"

"Maybe for both of us."

"'Cause feeling my physical boy-fat made you hot and bothered instead of a girl fantasy in your mind?"

"...To be honest, yeah."

"Don't get paranoid about it. Most males are hard-wired to like bods like mine. ...Hey, that's another pun."

"'Cause it's kind of a female shape?"

"That's the obvious interpretation; but it's also a baby shape, and most normal males feel protective of babies. But it causes conflict 'cause males in this society are taught that being fat is bad and feeling attracted to boys is wrong... 'specially if they're soft, warm and friendly. Conflict causes confusion, and people don't like feeling confused so they tend to hate what confuses 'em 'cause it's easier than figuring it out."

"I'll make a note of that," said Brandon.

Tommy smiled again. "You should never be scared of your own mind; just don't listen to *all* the voices."

"If you'd heard one of them a few seconds ago you might be the one who's scared."

"You should hear a few of mine."

"...Do any talk about me?"

"I don't wanna have to kill you." Tommy plopped back in the chair. "But, returning to research, I'm inside my fat, you're not. So you can't know how it feels to me. ...Like, petting a puppy feels good, but you don't know how it feels to have fur."

"How *does* it feel to you?" asked Brandon.

"I wish I could hug myself like you did and feel all my soft, warm friendliness."

"Would you hug another fat dude?"

"If he understood why."

"So he wouldn't get confused?"

"Are you confused anymore?"

"Not as much... but I'm not fat."

"But you're my friend, and that feels good, too."

"Like, on a different level?"

"I think we've made some progress today." Tommy looked back at the screen. "The coolest thing about our story is Beast is a cool young male who just happens to be fat."

Brandon smiled. "So is Tommy."

"Don't forget bitchin' and boss... the me I always wanted to be and you always thought I was. But I didn't know it myself at first... what we were doing with our site. Till we started getting all those posts saying we made fat kids feel good."

"Well, why should they feel bad?" said Brandon. "Feeling bad isn't healthy no matter what anyone weighs."

Tommy nodded. "One of the doctors told my mom that diets and dissing were stressing me out. Like, she was *trying* to make me unhealthy to prove that being fat was bad."

"What did she do?"

"Got a new doctor."

TEN

"Okay," said Brandon. "We built a fat-acceptance site, even if we didn't know it. What else is there in the fat universe?"

Tommy's fingers flew over the keys. "Here's a cool site with famous fat kids. Like, Joe Cobb and Norman Chaney from *The Little Rascals*. And Spanky, who was only a little chubby. Here's the dude who played Vern in *Stand By Me*, but he was only chubby, too. ...Did you notice the fat kid in the pie-eating contest was really wearing a padded suit?"

Brandon laughed. "You told me that a million times. ...And there's Larry Mondello."

"And here's all the dudes who played Pugsly Addams in the movies and on TV. Tim Weatherwax was the first, back in the 1960s. Pugsly is a boss fat kid who's not a stereotype. And there's Rerun from the *Right-on* show. And Game Boy and Gordon in *Way Past Cool*. And some fat kids from commercials... 'cept they don't use many fat kids. And never in fast-food commercials. And Brett Kelly in *Bad Santa*, and Julian Dennison in *Hunt for the Wilderpeople*."

Brandon again felt a twinge of something he'd felt in P.E. class today: there were *lots* things he would never be part of. "What else is there?"

"Tons of fat stuff! Chat rooms and forums where you can ask questions. From real doctors who don't hate fat kids. ...Like, how to deal with being dissed. And parents who put you on unhealthy diets. And brothers and sisters who who rag your ass till you wanna kill yourself. And how to deal with haters... like assholes down at the Boardwalk. And how to report teachers at school who make fat-hater

87

jokes or treat you mean. ...I got one of those this year. Then there's gainers, encouragers, admirers and feeders."

"Slow down, man," said Brandon. "For a fat kid you're really hyper."

"That's another stereotype... fat kids are slow and stupid."

"What's an encourager?"

"Someone who wants their friend to get fat. And/or fatter. Some encouragers are fat themselves, but others aren't and don't wanna be."

Brandon snagged his journal. "What's an admirer?"

"Someone who admires fat people. Like encouragers, sometimes they're fat, but mostly they're not."

"Who feeds the feeders?" asked Brandon.

"Feeders feed people who wanna get fed... feedees."

"To get fat and/or fatter?"

"Mostly," said Tommy. "But you can be both. Like, if two feeders hook up."

"To get fat and/or fatter together?" asked Brandon, rapidly scrawling more notes.

"Yeah," said Tommy. "You can do that in realtime, but a lot of kids do it in cyberspace. Same with admiring or encouraging." He smiled. "This could take a while, Brandon. I've been fat for twelve years and you never noticed."

"'Course I noticed."

"But it's like what Sherlock Holmes said: 'You look, but you do not see. ...Not till today, anyhow. So, what happened, Brandon? Did you have a near-fat experience? ...Besides just now with me."

"...Maybe I did," said Brandon. "But how come you never told me about all this fat stuff, Tommy? It's like an alternate universe. And it's like you're somebody else I never even knew."

"You could call it my Dark Side, Luke. ...If you thought it was bad."

"I *don't* think it's bad, I just feel left out. Like, you knew how to surf or play guitar but you never told me. ...What other secrets have you been keeping?"

"Had a major wet dream last night."

"Thanks for sharing. Anything else?"

"I could tell you the dream, but I'd have to kill you."

"Was I in it?"

"Then you'd kill me."

"You dream about me *that* way?"

"You weren't doing anything Bucky wouldn't do."

"Bucky can get pretty wild sometimes."

Tommy smiled. "Yeah, I know."

"You're in a lot of my dreams, too… and Beast can get pretty wild."

"I'm sure there's gonna be more now."

"It's your fault if there are."

"I doubt if you'll need therapy. …Hey, you got a message."

Brandon made a few more notes. "If it's BarbieGurl7, trash it."

"Thought you had the hots for her?"

"Not anymore. She went to our site and saw my pic. Said I wasn't ripped enough, but hit her up if I got in shape."

"That bitch is toast. But, this is from WoollyMammoth… that's a boss SN."

"He's one of the dudes I met today, and he's really fat."

"Which got you confused?"

"…To be honest, a little."

"Till you slapped yourself with sublimation."

"Which you explained, so I'm normal now."

"I'll bill you tomorrow." Tommy laughed. "You did have a near-fat experience."

"But, I like girls."

"I thought we got past that. Liking fat dudes doesn't mean you're gay. Just like Troy and his muscle-boy sites."

"Zot?"

"He admires ripped dudes but he's not gay."

"But, I like Travis… that's his name… because he's cool, not 'cause he's fat. The same way I like you."

"You just found more to like about me."

"…Well, yeah."

"If I may presume, you're wondering if every time we do it you're

89

gonna be thinking about my fat?"

"Or just seeing you in a different way."

"There's nothing wrong with the latter. And the former will soon become just an option 'cause you are basically normal."

"Only basically?" asked Brandon.

"If you were what passes for mainstream normal we wouldn't be having this conversation."

"That's lot of food for thought, especially for one meal." Then Brandon smiled. "Ask Travis to cam and you can admire."

"How do you know I'm an admirer?"

"You were educating Bucky, remember?"

"Houston, we have a problem. He doesn't have cam. No voice, neither."

"Either. Just read it the old-fashioned way."

"On screen. ...'Hey, Brandon? Wanna come over?'" Tommy turned to Brandon. "Can I come? Where's he live?"

"Down in The Flats."

"Da Beast lives for danger. ...Um, if you want me along?"

"We're Bucky and Beast, remember? Get up and let me answer."

"I'm too fat to get up. Help me."

"Get real."

"That used to be one of my fantasies. Getting so fat I couldn't walk. My mom woulda been soooo embarrassed."

"But how could you skate if you got that fat?"

"Were you logical when you were five?"

"Do some kids really get that fat?"

"There's some sites for immobile kids, but they're mostly older teens."

"And they're really too fat to walk?"

"Usually not totally, but not in the way we know it, Jim. Most of those kids are called immobile 'cause their thighs get so fat they can't walk very far. And it looks funny to haters, so they don't wanna be seen."

"Travis is kinda like that," said Brandon. "Except he's not scared of being seen."

"It's also hard to walk when your belly hangs down real far 'cause

90

you gotta keep shoving it out of your way."

"Travis is like that, too. It's hard for him to get up steps. But he's not embarrassed about that either. If he was he wouldn't be in that school. If people don't hate you for being fat, they hate you for some-thing else. It's like a public hate factory."

"Some really fat kids don't go to school. Just like there's an invisible web, there's also invisible fat kids."

"Do gainers want to get that fat?"

"For most of them it's a fantasy, even if they don't know it."

"Well, let's get the big fat Beast on his feet." Brandon slipped his hands under Tommy's arms and helped him out of the chair. "Woah, you're heavy!"

"Let's do it again and this time I won't help."

"So I can go back to the chiropractor?" Brandon settled at the keyboard, about to type a reply to Travis, but paused to ask, "Do you think I'm an admirer... but maybe in the closet? I always thought you looked cool."

Tommy laughed. "Thanks. But, do you think Zach looks cool?"

"In his own way."

"How about Chad?"

"Sure."

"And Troy?"

"As much as I hate to admit it."

Tommy laughed again. "You're not a fat admirer, you admire everybody for being who they are. ...How about yourself?"

Brandon looked into the full-length mirror mounted on his closet door. "There's not much to admire."

"Hey, Brandon, you're boss and bitchin'. ...Besides, a fat admirer would have noticed I gained twenty pounds this summer."

"An encourager would have encouraged you? And a feeder would have helped you get fatter?"

"See, it's not so complicated."

Brandon typed a reply. "Told him I'm bringing my homie. What's your curfew this year?"

"Ten on school nights unless I'm with you."

"Can you sleep over?"

"Sure. But mom wants me home for the starvation ration that currently passes for dinner."

"How long will that take? It's 6:03 now. I told Travis we'd be there at eight."

"How long does it take to eat half a grapefruit."

"Um, he's black."

"Cool," said Tommy. "Hence 'my homie.' ...I saw the *fattest* little black dude today! ...I'm talkin' PHAT in all caps! He was at the bus stop on Bay Street. Maybe only a sixth-grader, but man was he awesomely fat!"

"That's disgusting!" snapped a voice.

"Some people knock," said Tommy as Troy came in from the hall.

"Friends have keys, you fat tub of blubber."

"Then you musta stolen yours."

"'Fat tub of blubber' is redundant," said Brandon. "...What the mook happened to you?"

Troy glanced down at himself. He was wearing just sneaks and his school gym shorts, and panting for breath while dripping sweat. "Nothin's... the matter," he puffed. "I just... spent an hour workin' out, and... then I ran up... to the Bridges... and back."

Brandon laughed. "You look like that dude we chased on the beach. After we caught him."

"He wasn't... in shape," panted Troy. "All those... beaner kids... get obese."

"Which was probably lucky for us. I still have the scar where he bit me."

"You're lucky you had all your shots."

"You can tell him that," said Brandon. "I'll watch, it might be fun."

"What are you talking about?" puffed Troy, slowly regaining his breath.

"He's in our P.E. class this year. And he was the dude you dissed in the hall. He does speak English, *señor*."

"...Oh," said Troy.

Brandon offered the bottle. "Sorry I don't have another brew, but there's milk and OJ in the fridge."

"Thanks," said Troy. "But I'll just have some Calistoga. Beer has too many carbs. I gotta burn off this fat."

"What fat?" asked Tommy. "Your frontal lobes?"

"Shut up, you obese little pig!"

"Give it up, Troy," said Brandon. "You're never gonna look like Kelvin. He was designed that way and you're not. He doesn't even work out."

"Who's Kelvin?"

"The ripped black dude from P.E. class. The one you were admiring."

"...Well, like I said, it's natural with them. Which is kinda disgusting."

"No, it's good genes."

"If he had good genes he wouldn't be black. ...Did you shower with him?"

"...Oh yeah, man. Like, we washed each other all over and then rubbed down with warm baby oil."

"Bite me, Brandon, you know what I mean."

Brandon smiled. "He is a little bigger than you."

"So is a chipmunk," said Tommy.

"Shut up, fat-ass!" yelled Troy. He turned back to Brandon. "So, what's with this Special Ed shit? That's for obese kids an' retards. There's nothing wrong with you. ...Except you're a little retarded sometimes."

"It's my back," said Brandon, who didn't feel like explaining. "I hurt it trying to be something I'm not."

"Oh," said Troy. "I didn't know it was serious. But I get backaches all the time. No pain, no gain."

"No brain, no pain," said Tommy.

"Shut up, titty-boy!"

"Notice the Freudian slip," said Tommy.

"Noted," said Brandon.

"The hell you talking about?" Troy demanded.

"The answer is 42," said Tommy.

"It might be temporary," said Brandon. "Being in Special Ed."

"So, you're not stuck there? You can get back into normal P.E.?"

93

"Pesumably, if I wanted to."

Troy frowned. "If you meant 'something you're not' as in not being cool, you're right. You didn't *have* to hang with those losers after P.E. ...And how could you like them anyway? They can't be smart or they wouldn't be fat."

"I could resent that," said Tommy.

"I could hurt you, obese pig."

"You'd like that, wouldn't you?"

"I'd like to lock your fat ass in a cage! Like a naked obese little pig!"

"Mixed metaphor," said Brandon. "Rather retarded, actually."

Tommy turned to Brandon. "Also a common fixation for haters. To strip a fat kid naked and have him under control. The aspects of control and confinement, including control of appearance and weight, are also obsessions of most pedophiles... who generally tend to be fat-phobic and often fanatically so... but in this case I don't think we need to go there."

"Give it up, lardo," growled Troy. "You'll never be a psychiatrist. Who'd wanna go to a fat one?"

"Somebody who wanted to get well."

"Shut up, fatso!"

"You're right about that. I'm fat... so?"

"Maybe it's humiliation?" said Brandon.

Tommy spread his arms. "But I'm not humiliated when people see my boss fat bod." He grinned at Troy. "Perhaps you're simply in conflict between what you genuinely feel and what you've been taught you should feel?"

Troy stepped to Tommy. "Shut up, or...!"

"Leave him alone," said Brandon. "Or I might have to hurt you."

"Like you could, you marshmallow wimp!"

"Hmm," said Brandon. "'Losers' did you say? Including Bosco Donatello, whose autographed picture is no doubt hanging on your bedroom wall at this very moment."

"He's a good surfer, he's just too fat."

"To be a good surfer?" asked Tommy.

"Quit trying to confuse me, you little fat-ass!"

"You don't need my help with that."

Brandon shook his head. "You're really being a mook today, Troy. ...You want what's left of this beer or not?"

"I guess." Troy took the bottle and sucked it dry. "Can I use your sauna?"

"If you promise not to melt in there like the Wicked Witch of the West. Set the timer in case you pass out."

"I'm in the best shape I've ever been in! Look at me, dammit!" Troy flexed his arms and puffed his chest.

Brandon sighed. "It's the shape of your mind that worries me."

"It's called growing up, you should try it sometime." Troy opened the sliding glass door that overlooked the swimming pool and the sauna house beside it. "Wanna shoot hoops later on?"

"Tommy and me are going out."

"Tommy and I," said Tommy.

Troy snorted. "Why don't you dress him up like a girl so people would think you could actually get one."

"His slip is showing again," said Tommy.

Troy scowled. "Why are you two always shirtless together? That's starting to look really gay."

"Then put one on," said Brandon. "And we've all been swimming naked since we were little kids."

"Nor did you seem to think," added Tommy, "that pounding your pony with us was gay... to use the clinical term."

"I stopped doing that last month; it drains your physical energy."

"Which might explain your pent-up frustrations."

Brandon laughed. "Bet you've been having some record wet dreams."

"We're not little kids anymore!" snapped Troy. "At least I'm not!"

"Your anxieties and inhibitions are developing right on schedule," said Tommy.

"Your tits are already way too developed!"

"That's three slips," said Tommy.

"The answer is 42," said Brandon.

Troy shook his head. "I don't know which one of you is more mooked up, Tommy for getting so freakin' obese..." He shifted his eyes to Brandon. "Or you for being his friend. ...The hell you see in him anyway? Lots of people think you're weird for hanging with him all the time."

"I must be weird. Look at the shit I put up with from you."

"Grow the fuck up!"

"When they tell you to shut up, they mean stop talking."

"Whatever," said Troy, stalking out and slamming the door.

"Sorry, Tommy," said Brandon. "Maybe it's just his time of the month."

"It's cool, Brandon, I'm used to it."

"Chad calls you lots of names, too."

"It's different with him," said Tommy. "He doesn't really know what he's saying. It's just hater stuff he's heard on TV. He's not trying to hurt me."

"But, Troy is?"

"I don't think we've lost him yet. I'd say he still thinks he's trying to help me... dropping tough love on the poor obese kid to make him wanna lose weight."

"It still sucks."

Tommy shrugged. "The strong survive, and they come in all sizes."

Brandon's phone rang on the bedside table. "Hello? ...Hi, dad. What's up?"

Another phone beeped.

"Zot?" said Tommy, looking around.

"In my pack," said Brandon. "...No, dad, it's my wireless. Wait." Brandon took his new phone from Tommy. "Hello? ...Hi, mom." He put a phone to each ear. "...Oh. that sucks... You too, dad? Oh, that sucks.. ...No, dad, she's right here... No, mom, he's right here. ...Wait a second." Brandon held the phones together and grinned at Tommy. "It's mom and dad."

"Who woulda guessed."

"There was another wreck on the summit. They're both stuck in traffic," said Brandon. "Mom said to order dinner, so I'll get you one, too."

Another phone rang in the kitchen.

"Get that, Beast," said Brandon.

"On it, Bucky."

"Huh?" Brandon said to the phones. "It's Tommy, he's sleeping over tonight. ...Yeah, mom, he told me what his mom said. ...No, I won't let him eat anything. He can sit here and watch me stuff my face. ...Yeah, not funny. ...Yeah, 'obese.' ...Ten years off his life, yeah. ...School was okay, dad. Writing class rocks! ...So, what's my curfew this year? I wanna go see a friend. ...Eleven is okay, I guess. ...Not very enthusiastic? If I got all hot and wet about it you'd think you were being too liberal. ...Sorry. ...Yeah, it's cool you trust me."

Tommy returned from the kitchen. "It was my mom." He stuck a finger down his throat. "Diet time, back in five. Tell Mobile Meals to use warp nine."

"See ya," said Brandon. "...No, mom, dad, that was Tommy. Chad went out somewhere. Want me to search his room for meth and automatic weapons?"

"Wanna die painfully?" asked Chad, coming in from the hall, his own phone to an ear. "Who the mook are you talking to?"

"Mom and dad," said Brandon. "They're stuck on the summit again. ...Here." He shoved the phones at his brother.

"Dork!" said Chad, juggling phones. "...No, not you, Lisa."

97

ELEVEN

"**M**an I'm stuffed!" panted Tommy, gently massaging his middle while stopping his board by dragging a sneak. He was still clad in his cutoffs, but also a 'beater so small and tight that most of his belly was hanging bare while his breasts bobbled out on each side. "That was a bitchin' dinner! I *almost* couldn't eat it all, which would have been a first for me."

"You're taking ten years off your life," puffed Brandon, who was wearing a black tank-top and a pair of his newest jeans. The night was warm and the boys were sweating, though the ride had been mostly downhill.

"Based on whose research?" asked Tommy.

Brandon shrugged. "Mom said that on the phone when she told me not to feed you tonight."

Tommy burped for the millionth time since they'd kicked away from Brandon's house, rolling along the asphalt path that hugged the West Cliff shoreline and past the lighthouse on the Point. "Even if that was true... which has not been objectively proven... that's ten years off the *end* of my life, which is usually mookie anyhow. Ask my grand-father in Golden Years Home when he's getting his diaper changed. ...And if you want some medical *fact* instead of junk science and biased conjecture, I'm healthier than a lot of skinny kids. Really pisses my doctor off... the new fat-hater one... 'cause he can't find anything wrong with me. All he can say is I'm fat."

"I thought the new word was obese?" said Brandon.

"'Cause it sounds a lot worse than just fat. Like, saying 'using alcohol' instead of just drinking beer."

98

"But, what if you get too fat?" asked Brandon.

"By whose definition?"

"...Well... by yours, since it's your body."

"As long as I'm happy being me, I'll never be too fat."

"Maybe I'm an encourager? I didn't have to buy you all that."

"Do you want me to get fatter?"

"That's not a yes or no question."

"I'll rephrase," said Tommy. "Would you still be my friend if I lost weight?"

"As long as you were still you."

"'Cool, smart, and fun to be with?'"

"Don't forget bitchin' and boss."

"Then you're not an encourager. You aren't trying to make me get fatter, and you'd still like me if I lost weight."

"An encourager isn't really a friend."

"Care to expand on that?"

"It's liking somebody for what's on the outside. For how they look, not who they are. That's not being a friend, at least by my definition."

"In many cases that's true," said Tommy. "But why did you like that girl today? The one you saw at school."

"...Well... she was pretty. But, like I said, she also looked smart."

"Would you encourage her to read books to make her smarter because you like smart?"

"Guess I would," said Brandon.

"You also said she was charmingly chubby, something else you obviously liked."

"You mean would I encourage her to get a little chubbier? I never thought about things like that."

"Then you're not an encourager."

"So, maybe I'm an enabler 'cause I gave you all that food?"

"Where did you come up with that one?"

"Mom said it on the phone tonight in reference to not feeding you."

"She probably got it from my mom, who got it from my new doctor. There's a stupidity epidemic and it's very viral. But, it's normal to have a preference for a physical shape, and to want to enhance what you like. I encouraged Zach this summer."

Brandon laughed. "I don't think he needs much encouraging. You should have seen him at lunch today. Got me to buy him a whole bunch of food after he spent all his money. He ate more than the really fat dudes. ...Are you saying I encouraged a gainer?"

"I think we could go with 'enabled' in that case. and unintentionally... unless knowing you were making him fatter gave you gratification."

"I get it," said Brandon. "And if I may venture a layman's opinion, judging from all his stretch marks, he obviously got triggered this summer."

"Bucky does catch on fast."

"But I don't get the trigger part. You trigger a gun to shoot it, but it has to be loaded."

"Go with that," said Tommy. "It's a good metaphor."

"...Well... a gun has to have bullets to shoot. Which means there has to be something inside."

"And a gun can be loaded for years," said Tommy. "Call it being dormant until something triggers it. As related to the subject at hand, it's usually loaded in childhood, and often on a subconscious level, by something experienced, seen or heard. The process is totally normal, and often influences our future... what we want to do, how we want to look, and a lot of the choices we make in life, including what kind of people we like."

"So, Zach saw a fat kid when he was little and thought it was cool, which 'loaded' him, and something pulled his trigger last summer, so now he wants to get fat?"

"It could be that simple," said Tommy. "But I try not to analyze my friends."

"That must be like having X-ray vision but being too polite to use it."

Tommy shrugged. "Most fortune-tellers can analyze people more accurately than psychiatrists. ...You'll be killed if you tell anybody."

"How come you didn't wear something cooler? Clothes are important to black kids."

"They're not important to white ones?"

"You had that shirt in sixth grade and you barely fit into it then."

"I'm meeting your school's fattest kid," said Tommy. "Don't want him to think I'm a hider."

"Hider?"

"Fat kids who wear oversize clothes to try to hide their fat. Some even wear special underwear to conceal their contours, 'specially if they have boy-breasts."

"Because they're ashamed of their fat?"

"Some are, but others like being fat and just don't wanna get dissed. ...I assume Travis isn't a hider?"

Brandon laughed. "Anything but! You should have seen him in P.E. today. And none of the other fat dudes were shy, except this skeezer, Jason."

"There's always a Jason to mook up our image. ...So, who's this 'loser?' The one who Troy got a picture of?"

"Bosco Donatello. And he's not a loser in any sense."

"Sounds like you met a lot of cool dudes."

"I'm up to my ass in cool dudes this year. ...That sounded like a Freudian slip."

"Sometimes an ass is just an ass."

"Which is a first for me. Now if I could just meet a cool girl."

"Which would also be a first."

"Thanks, doctor, I needed that."

Tommy scanned the gloomy street. "Spooky as mook with the Boardwalk closed."

"Yeah," agreed Brandon, looking around. "Reminds me of that *Lost Boys* movie they made down here a long time ago."

The Flats was composed of a few small blocks along the Santa Cruz Boardwalk. It lay within a loop of levee where the San Lorenzo River ran to meet the sea at the beach. The houses were mostly small bungalows that had once been summer retreats for the rich; and here and there were old motels -- the Surf & Sun, the Sea & Sand -- with rooms including "kitchenettes" that overflowed with families who weren't there on vacation.

There were also a few Victorian houses, like smaller, shabbier poor relations of grander homes atop Beach Hill. The buildings down here were crowded together as if they'd all been rounded up, imprisoned behind the river wall and told they'd be shot if they tried to leave.

The narrow streets were more like alleys and laid out like a labyrinth with many dead-ends and confusing turns. The lamps were few and far between, and only seemed to annoy the dark. Sneaker fruit dangled from telephone wires, and this season's crop was abundant.

The Boardwalk lay along Beach Street between the wharf and the river mouth, its lofty rides and roller-coaster looming against the starry sky. But the place looked strange and creepy tonight, the rides shut down, their lights all out; eerily dead without the crowds, the music from the merry-go-round, and the rattle and roar of coaster cars. Brandon would have written: *like an abandoned factory where fun had once been made.*

A few figures haunted the shadowy streets here in the darkest heart of The Flats. Many were kids who seemed to be searching for some-thing recently lost... the music, lights, and bright arcades that had given them refuge all summer. The Boardwalk had also provided free meals, when tourists left their picnic baskets unattended on the beach, or burgers and fries alone on tables while getting extra condiments. The local word was "gulling," and Brandon and Tommy had gulled a few times just for the fun of feeding themselves on somebody else's food. It was funny to see their victims' faces after the grub had disap-peared... why would anyone steal a meal? Wallets, watches, purses, yes; but why would anyone jack their *food* in the richest nation on earth?

Skaters occasionally rattled past on battered boards with worn out wheels, and none of the kids on rusty bikes were wearing safety helmets. The fine was fifty dollars, which Brandon's parents had paid a few times. He wondered what happened to these kids... were they thrown in jail for not being safe if they couldn't afford to pay for their safety?

He'd also seen a lot of fat kids, proportionally more than in wealthier 'hoods. That might have been a lucky thing because he'd spotted a possible ambush in front of a liquor store; three boys who seemed to be waiting for prey. But two of the dudes were as fat as Carlos and stepped aside as Tommy rolled by, returning his "s'up" with "lookin' good."

"Is that a fat brotherhood thing?" Brandon had asked, after they'd left the boys behind.

"Sometimes," Tommy had replied, "but I've been jacked by XXLs. Fat kids can be bad like anyone else."

Now, Brandon peered at a sign on a pole, rusty and barely readable. "This is the street. ...Must be that house over there. Travis said he'd turn on the porch light."

The house was a narrow two-stories tall, one of the shabby Victorians with a tiny patch of yard. The lawn was mostly crab-grass, a thing of shame to Brandon's dad, but here neatly trimmed and bordered with flowers. The house's roof was sagging a bit, and the front porch steps looked rotten. A floor lamp shone through faded shades in what must have been the living room, and a light bulb burn-ed in a second-floor window, showcasing cracks in a plaster ceiling.

Toting their boards under their arms, the boys came up the buckled walk, but Tommy paused to sniff the air. "I smell barbecued ribs. Mmmm."

"Shut up!" snapped Brandon.

"Zot?"

"That's not funny, Tommy! Especially from someone who lectur-ed me about stereotyping people."

"But I *do* smell ribs," said Tommy. "Is there something wrong with your nose?"

"I smell 'em, too," said Brandon, as if admitting to something.

"Can't black people eat ribs?" asked Tommy. "That's a stereotype in reverse. Politically-correct paranoia. ...And, I had ribs on Wednesday night."

"I had 'em the other night, too," said Brandon. "But, don't say anything about 'em."

"I had fried chicken on Friday."

"Shut up."

103

The steps cried out like tortured souls as Tommy and Brandon ascended. The porch creaked loudly underfoot; and Brandon had to remind himself that Travis trod these ancient planks and obviously hadn't broken through. The bell button didn't look functional but Brandon pushed it anyhow. He was almost surprised to hear a buzz above the sound of a television... a Burger King commercial. The scent of ribs was enticing his nose, though his belly was too stuffed to growl. Floorboards popped and squeaked in the house as someone heavy approached.

"Sounds like my kinda dude," whispered Tommy.

The hinges gave a ghastly screech as a black kid opened the door. Aromatic heat poured out, steamy-rich and meaty delicious, but Bran-don almost gaped in shock. A weird thought flashed through his mind... Travis White had been cloned!

The boy was maybe eleven but must have weighed over 300 pounds. He was wearing only white boxer shorts, which were barely visible because of a massively mammoth belly that hung all the way to his chub-padded knees. Like Travis' belly, its bottom half was a pendulous pair of tear-drop shapes with a funnel-like cave of a navel tunneling deeply upward between; and he looked like a lesson in drawing cartoons where everything was an oval or sphere, from the bulbously bulging balloons of his chest, which were easily twice the size of Tommy's, to a bottom like ebony moons colliding and barely contained by his sagging shorts, which carelessly clung to his blubber-bulked thighs. Like Travis, he jiggled and quivered all over with even the slightest move.

"Hey, man!" said Tommy. "I saw you on Bay Street today. You're mad wicked totally cool! I'm Tommy."

"Hey," said the mammoth little boy. "You're mad wicked crazy cool. I'm Ro."

"You are *awesome*, man!"

Ro grinned. "Back at ya. Want some ribs?"

"Def!"

Ro offered a rib he was holding. "I didn't bite it yet."

"I wouldn't care," said Tommy, accepting it with reverence.

"I wanna get me a board," said Ro, checking Tommy's plank.

104

"I could help you learn to ride."

"Cool," said Ro. "Want some more ribs? All you can eat."

"Those last four words are my favorites," said Tommy, around a mouthful of meat."

"Um..." said Brandon. Feeling a little left-out again because of the fat kid camaraderie. "We came to see Travis."

"He's up in our room," said Ro, pointing to a steep, narrow staircase.

"Roosevelt?" called a woman's voice from what was probably the kitchen. "Who's there, honey?"

"Travis's friends. Gonna give 'em some ribs."

A man's voice called, "Give 'em a lot more than some!"

It wasn't a total surprise to Brandon that Travis's mother was huge: it did seem kind of logical. Could a smiling sun be black, he wondered? Maybe an ebony star? She filled the kitchen doorway, beaming a welcome into the room. "Hello, boys. I hope you're hungry."

"Hi, Mrs. White," said Brandon, thinking of oxymorons.

A man looked over the woman's shoulder. He was also fat, and darker than Travis... which Brandon found amazing. He was wearing a sweaty T-shirt, and a white cotton cap like a cook's. He chuckled like Travis:" Don't be shy, food's for eating."

"Um," said Brandon. "Thank you, sir."

The woman nudged the man. "Told you our boys always pick good friends. ...Which one of you is Brandon?"

"Him," said Tommy. "I'm Tommy Turner."

"Brandon Williams," said Brandon.

"Nice to meet you," said the man. "I'm Rick and this is Sherry. Travis is up in his room."

"Our room," Ro corrected.

"Right up those stairs," said Sherry.

"I already told 'em," said Ro. "Tommy's gonna teach me skatin' soon's I get a board."

"Save your money," said the man. "Soon as you start making some."

Roosevelt turned to Tommy. "Y'all go on up, I'll bring you some food."

"You're so *phat!*" said Tommy, the spelling sounding obvious.

"I know." Roosevelt rippled and wobbled away, sort of kneeing his belly along and waddling like a penguin, and Tommy headed for the stairs across the living room. "My mom would have apologized."

"For what?" asked Brandon.

"For having a fat kid, duh. Instead of saying I get good grades or read lots of books, she would have said, 'he's on a diet.' Or 'he's going on one.' Like everybody wants to know about my 'weight problem.'"

"That's gotta suck."

"Like a black hole, and that's not a Freudian slip."

Brandon looked around the room as they reached the foot of the stairs. He got the impression of lively clutter, of things well-worn and used a lot; a sofa, big chairs, a colorful carpet, a tasseled floor lamp, an ancient TV. The dark-paneled walls were adorned with pictures, probably Travis's family, and most of them were fat. There were also a few from Black History Month; Dr. Martin Luther King, Malcolm X. Was that Huey Newton? A McDonalds commercial was on the TV, happy children stuffing their faces while Ronald McDonald encouraged them.

Brandon paused to watch. There were no fat kids in those commercials, or even chubby ones.

"That's the new Extra Happy Meal," said Tommy. "Everything super-size."

The house had a homey kind of smell, food and cooking -- especially ribs -- soap in a sink, shampoo in a shower, and more than a hint of sweaty boys. The windows all seemed to be open, but the heat inside was intense.

"You have to eat that," Brandon whispered, as he and Tommy climbed the stairs, which squeaked and creaked under Tommy's tread. "It's not polite to refuse food in anybody's culture."

"I'm the politest dude on the planet. ...And it rocks! Killer sauce! Here, take a chomp."

"Its good," agreed Brandon, taking a nibble. "But, I'm gonna explode if I eat any more."

"Looks like you're gonna have to. It's not polite to refuse food in anybody's culture."

TWELVE

Despite its lofty Victorian ceilings, the place looked like a doll house to Brandon as they reached the top of the stairs; like something Disney had built for kids and then forgotten a long time ago. The hall was taller than it was wide, and the floor was sagging cartoonishly, which seemed to have slanted the walls. There were three doorways, one showing light... the unfrosted glow in the second-floor window Brandon had seen from the street. He paused for a moment to peep inside before lifting a hand to knock, though it seemed silly to bother with knocking since Travis was sitting just ten feet away facing a little CRT screen, his fingers busily clattering keys. He apparently knew how to touch-type, and worked at warp-nine compared to Brandon. He was seated beside the open window, black as the night in just snowy white shorts, and seemingly crushing an old swivel chair. He'd looked enormous in school today, but seemed even fatter in this tiny space, which was smaller than Brando's bathroom.

Travis's desk was an old kitchen table, so piled with books and other stuff that his ancient computer was almost buried. The light bulb dangled from dangerous wires, and homemade book shelves lined the walls. There were toys and action-figures – probably Roosevelt's -- scattered around, while every square inch of free wall space was plastered with drawings and pictures.

Magazines covered the bare board floor like a colorful carpet of graphics. Many were manga and anime, while others featured classic cartoons. Brandon noticed *Heavy Metal* along with *Mad* and comic books, but there was also serious stuff like *Rolling Stone* and *Mother Jones*. There was *Psychology Today* -- which Tommy also subscribed to -- and several other cerebral journals that dealt with health and science. These seemed to balance fantasy, gothic, ghosts, and horror.

The books on the shelves were wildly eclectic, from John Steinbeck and J.D. Salinger, to works by Edgar Allen Poe. Herman Melville shared a shelf with H.P. Lovecraft and Larry Niven. Bram Stoker nudged Ralph Ellison, while J.R.R. Tolkien met Kurt Vonnegut, who chilled with Jonathan Swift. A complete set of *Elfquest* stood side-by-side with Charles Dickens and Thorne Smith, while Dr. Suess elbowed Dr. Ruth in a mix of Mark Twain and Hunter S. Thompson. Many volumes were ancient hardcovers bound in cloth or leather. Several looked like magic books that might have been found in a wizard's lair, while others appeared to be medical texts like Brandon had seen in his doctor's office.

Half the room was taken up by a double-size mattress that lay on the floor. It was messily made with rumpled blankets and feral leopard-pattern sheets. There was also a ramshackle dresser, plastered with decals and stickers, and painted screaming yellow. A battered blaster sat on top, bumping out *Time For Me To Fly*, a classic rock song by REO Speedwagon.

"Woah," said Brandon. "This place is boss!"

"With a bitchin' bullet!" said Tommy.

Travis had turned at the sound of their voices, his old chair scream-ing as loud as the dresser. "C'mon in."

"Oh man!" said Tommy, gazing at Travis as if he'd found the Holy Grail. "You're way too past cool for this universe!"

Brandon murmured, "Chill out, Tommy."

"I can't help it. I wanna bow down!"

"Can if you want," said Travis, then laughed when Tommy dropped to his knees. "Sorry I don't have a ring to kiss. ...Make yourselves at home. Sorry it's hotter than hell up here, but my folks been cooking all day. Lose your shirts before you melt."

Tommy leaned his board against the wall and wiggled out of his 'beater.

"It'll probably last till Wednesday," said Brandon. "The warm weather, I mean." He stood his board next to Tommy's and pulled off his sweaty tank-top. "Then there'll be fog again for a week. But

109

there's always an Indian Summer. It was so hot one Halloween I went Trick-or-Treating as Mowgli."

"Naked?" asked Travis.

"Just a loincloth."

"Mowgli was raised by wolves," said Travis. "So, where did he get the loincloth? Did Mother Wolf knit it for him?"

"It's in the Disney movie," said Tommy. "But I never thought of that."

"Check out that book over there," said Travis. "Mowgli probably looked like him... a whole lot darker than Disney wanted. Probably a Tamil. And without the red diaper."

Tommy paged a tattered *Jungle Book*. "That's how I would have imagined him if Disney hadn't got to me first."

"But, some years it rains," Brandon added lamely, not knowing what else to say. Tommy and Travis, like Tommy and Ro, already seemed tight just because they were fat. "How long have you been in Santa Cruz?"

"Since school let out in June," said Travis. "We moved down here from Oakland after my folks got the fish 'n chips place." He grinned at Tommy, who'd returned the book to the shelf and was unabashedly scanning him as if to paint a portrait. "Look all you want, man, I won't charge."

"You're so mad phat!"

"Don't have an orgasm," said Brandon.

Travis laughed. "It's just a fat thing."

"So I've started to notice," said Brandon.

"He's down with us," said Tommy.

"So I've noticed," said Travis. "Kelvin went to the market for sodas. He should be back any minute."

"No forties?" asked Tommy.

"Maaan!" muttered Brandon.

"I didn't think about brew," said Travis.

"That's cool," said Brandon.

"What do you drink?"

"Mostly whatever my 'rents bring home... Heinekin, Lowenbrau, San Miguel. Even white wine if I'm desperate."

110

"Hey," said Tommy. "You do these cartoons? They're crazy boss!"

Brandon regarded the many drawings tacked or taped to the walls. Most were the same sort of Bambi-eyed boys that Travis had drawn on his binder. Many were fat or chubby, and most were black and looking cool, though Travis also drew cool white kids. ...Or maybe the term was "non-black kids?"

"Hey, this one's Ro," said Tommy. "You really drew him phat!"

Brandon laughed at a cartoon portrayal of Ro boasting breasts like black basketballs and a belly hanging down to his feet. "Was that your little-kid fantasy, Tommy?"

"When I started fighting mom." Tommy turned to Travis. "I assume you and Ro don't have that problem?"

"We never made it a problem," said Travis. "But, a lot of kids at Ro's school are haters. The teacher even dissed him right in front of the class. Used him for an example of 'morbidly obese.' Put the other kids against him. They gave him shit at recess. He's never had to deal with that."

"I think I got that teacher," said Tommy. "I'm gonna report her tomorrow."

"Think it'll do any good?" asked Travis. "Nobody cares if you dis fat kids."

"I'll email the A.C. L. U. if I have to."

"Maybe I will, too," said Travis. "This is the first time Ro's had to fight just because he's fat. He gave some hater a smack-down today, which got more respect than the teacher's hate shit."

"Don't they dis fat kids in Oakland?" asked Brandon. "...Um... other black kids, I mean."

"Nothing like assholes do here. We make fat jokes but it's not hate. Here, it's hate with a bullet." Travis leaned back in the creaky chair. "But, on to happy topics... we're having a kind of party tonight. My folks always wanted a rib shop. They've both been cooks for most of their lives. But all we could afford this year was the fish 'n chips booth at the Boardwalk. Mom buys fish fresh off the wharf, and Dad makes his own beer batter. The paper ran a story..." He pointed to a news-paper clipping taped above his computer. "'Best Fish 'N Chips On Monterey Bay.' We made good money this summer and got a loan from a bank, so we're getting a shop of our own next week."

"Cool," said Brandon. "I love ribs."

"Maaaan!" said Tommy.

"Oh, shut up."

Travis went on, "Mom and dad been cooking all day, trying out all their recipes and getting the neighbor's opinions. Now we're gonna eat what's left. There's beef and pork ribs, potato salad, cole slaw, beans and collards. Hope you dudes came hungry."

"...Oh," said Brandon. "That's really phat. But I don't know how much I can eat."

"Just concentrate on the ribs," said Travis.

"...Sure," said Brandon, who felt almost trapped. It was kind of like when he'd been ten, hanging with some friends from school who'd offered him a blunt: should he be cool and smoke, just say no like it said on TV, or make a lame excuse and go home?

Travis smiled. "Ro can eat a ton by himself. So can Kelvin. I hooked with Zach online and he's coming over, too."

"What about Carlos?" asked Brandon. "I'm sure he could eat a lot."

"Zach said he'd give him a call. His mom knows Carlos's mom from work. And I sent Danny an email." Travis glanced out the window. "There's Zach and Carlos now." He slowly unloaded his bulk from the chair, all his rolls rearranging themselves and his belly blubber a mid-night cascade – as Brandon would have written it -- the floor creaking loudly beneath his bare feet. "I'll help Ro with the plates; and Kel should be back with the drinks pretty soon. Check out my computer if you want, but file the story first, okay?" He lumbered into the hall, and the house seemed to shake as he went down the stairs one ponderous tread at a time.

Tommy regarded the monitor. "Last time I saw a Mac this old was in an antique shop."

"Guess they're kinda poor," said Brandon, looking around the tiny room. Lath peeked in places where plaster had fallen, and cracks etched the ceiling like old people's wrinkles.

Tommy laughed. "Travis and Ro are too phat to be rich. Money can't buy a room like this! ...Check this out. It's like the stories you

112

write... 'Bobby woke up to the sound of surf...'"

"That's not cool," said Brandon. "Never read a work in progress unless the writer invites you to."

"Oh. Sorry."

"File it like he said. ...You know how to work an old Mac?"

"Also a rotary phone."

Despite himself, Brandon read a few lines. It was a good beginning, using what Bosco had said that morning... waking up on a beach at dawn with the sun all rosy and gold on the water. Like being born again. Then he heard voices below, recognizing Carlos and Zach's as Roosevelt greeted them. Then the stairs began to creak.

"Yo, Brandon. ...Tommy!" Zach came in with two heaping plates, one piled high with juicy ribs, the other loaded with all the extras... a mountain of chunky potato salad laced with bits of onion and pickle, a towering mound of creamy cole slaw, and a fragrant heap of steaming greens. He was dressed the same as he'd been at school -- ancient Skunk jeans and the camouflage tee -- and was just about to lose the jeans since both his hands were occupied and his spherical belly bobbing part bare while far overhanging their half-buttoned fly. He paused for a second to scan around. "Killer location! ...Hey, Brandon, hold these." He handed the plates to Brandon, then stripped off his shirt and plopped on the mattress.

Carlos came in also carrying plates as Brandon returned Zach's food.

"Hey, Carlos," said Brandon. "This's Tommy."

"Yo, Tommy," said Carlos. "I seen you around the Boardwalk, man." He shed his shirt and sat down beside Zach. "Damn, man! There goes my zipper!" He hoisted two handfuls of belly fat and leaned way over to peer underneath. "I knew that was comin'!"

"Yeah," said Tommy. "After you lose the button on top, the zipper don't last very long."

"I noticed that, man," said Carlos. "Hey, Brandon, I sell you these Tommys cheap."

Zach laughed. "They might just fit him later, after we eat all this!"

"These jeans are new," said Brandon. "Thirty-two waist, plenty of

113

room."

"I'm up to thirty-four," said Zach. "'Course, that's way under my belly. I get my jeans at the Salvation Army. When you're gaining, new clothes are a waste of money better spent on food."

"Guess you'll lose your softee supply when the Boardwalk closes for winter." said Brandon.

"Yeah, but that's no problem. My girlfriend loves to feed me."

"Cool you got a... feeder," said Brandon, sitting down on the mattress.

Tommy landed beside him and smiled like an approving mentor. "Had a cute feeder, maybe thirteen, follow me from Pirate's Cove all the way to the Cave Train last week."

"What happened?" asked Zach.

"She was gonna buy me a burger and shake, but then her 'rents showed up. And they gave her that look... confused and pissed... like they'd seen her with fat dudes before."

"I know that look," said Zach. "I see it on a lotta 'rents when they see their kids admiring me." He turned to Brandon. "You a gainer?"

"...I gained a few pounds this summer."

Zach patted Brandon's tummy. "You need to gain more if you want admirers. Nikki Barnes, my girlfriend, wouldn't even look at me back when I was skinny."

"But, you must have looked something like me," said Brandon. "Before you put on weight. I wouldn't call that skinny."

"No offense," said Zach. "But there's billions of dudes who look like you. Nikki says they're boring. Like, who wants a boyfriend who looks like a clone of all the pretty boy-toys on TV?"

"Hey," said Tommy. "Brandon's one of a kind, even if he don't look it."

"Nothin' personal, Brandon," said Zach. "But I think you know what I mean. Like that *Twilight Zone* episode: 'Number Twelve Looks Just Like You.'"

"No prob," said Brandon. "And I kinda noticed that."

Carlos said, "A lot of our girls think fat dudes are phat. Like, it shows we're makin' it, man. You Anglos got the biggest prob with all that body image bull. Like, you made Barbie an' Ken into gods. Like

114

some sorta skinny-ass master race. An' you're tryin' to teach that to our little kids. ...That's a generic 'you,' man."

"I'm starting to notice that, too," said Brandon.

THIRTEEN

The staircase groaned and creaked again in a series of slowly ascending treads, and Travis and Ro waddled in from the hall, both bearing plates overflowing with food. "Here you go," panted Travis, handing helpings to Tommy and Brandon.

Again the stairs got vocal, and Danny appeared behind Ro, wearing dangerous jeans and a red T-shirt that couldn't cover his belly. His long raven hair was tamed by a band, and his chubby face gleamed like polished copper. He also toted a brimming plate. "Looks like a pow-wow in here."

"An' it's multicultural," said Carlos.

The little room was stuffed to bursting as Danny wiggled out of his shirt and joined the massive mosh on the mattress. Brandon glanced at the ancient floor, which seemed to be sagging ominously. He pictured it suddenly giving way and dumping them all in the basement. Maybe the newspaper headlines would read:

NEW DANGER IN CHILDHOOD OBESITY!
OBESE BOYS CAUSE HOUSE COLLAPSE!

Even with the window open the temperature was rising fast from all the sweaty bodies. The mattress seemed like a little life-raft adrift on a sea of magazines. Brandon was squeezed between Tommy and Zach, while Ro used Brandon's legs for a back rest. Brandon's back was pressed to Travis, which felt like a soft and slippery couch.

Propping the plate on his up-drawn knees, Brandon took a bite of rib and suddenly wanted to eat the whole thing despite being

116

stuffed from dinner. The meat was perfect in texture and taste, tender, and dripping with succulent juice, while the sauce was tangy, smoky and sweet. He'd thought he'd have to force himself, but the rib was a bone in seconds. He forked up a mound of potato salad. Everything tasted so mookin' good!

Was that because everyone else was eating... and without civilized manners? The mutant boys of Beastworld would probably feast like this, he thought. He made a mental note of that to use in a future episode.

The stairs squeaked softly and Kelvin appeared, a shirtless boy-god of pure midnight -- assuming a worship of muscular boys -- in faded jeans showing snowy shorts. He toted an armload of two-liter bottles along with a heaping plate. "Got Coke an' Sprite, root beer an' cherry, grape, cream soda, an' orange."

The other boys made room for him, though there was little to spare.

"Yo, Kel," said Travis. "This is Tommy, Brandon's BF."

"Yo, Tommy," said Kelvin.

"Mm," muffed Tommy. "Mah-mouff-fuh."

"Open the bottles and pass 'em," said Travis. "Any you guys got germs?"

"I had all my shots," said Danny and laughed. "Except the anti-fat vaccine."

"Is there one?" asked Brandon.

Travis said, "Some company's probably working on one. They won't help starving Africans, but they'll spend billions researching ways to make Americans skinny."

"While making trillions," said Tommy.

"Somebody turn up the tunes," said Carlos.

"Somebody skinny do it," said Ro. "I'm too fat to keep getting up."

"The skinny dude's buried in fat ones," laughed Brandon.

"I'll do it," said Kelvin.

"I think the beef ribs are better," said Ro.

"Tell that to dad," said Travis. "I dare you."

"The pork rocks, too," said Zach, his cheeks bulging round like a chipmunk's.

"There's different sauces," said Ro. "Check this one."

"Boss potato salad," said Tommy.

Brandon wasn't sure when things began to get confused. He'd planned to eat whatever he could to be polite to Travis, but the more he ate the more he wanted! That had never happened before. He'd never forced himself to eat, except the usual little-kid thing about "cleaning your plate before dessert," as if dessert was a sweet reward for eating things you didn't like. The same applied to Thanksgiving dinners when he'd been encouraged to stuff himself to show his gratitude to God. But everything tasted so mookin' good! It didn't seem fair that his stomach was stuffed and pleading with him to stop. ...But part of this pleasure *was* being stuffed.

It was sort of like getting drunk, when you'd passed beyond a happy buzz that merely made you feel good and wanted to reach a peaceful place where nothing mattered and time stood still. He'd also done that on dope, but stuffing his belly seemed a lot better; a happy, hazy, careless high.

Nothing around him was clear anymore; the bare light bulb a distant sun. He remembered his first time getting drunk with Troy on a summer afternoon. They had skated two sixers of Heinekin down to Santa Cruz Beach and started drinking under the wharf, careful at first and watching for cops. The Boardwalk had been crowded that day, teeming with tourists and swarming with vallies. Tanning oil and sunscreen fumes had filled the sultry air. But no one seemed to want to hassle a pair of drunken ten-year-olds... "the bad skate-punks from the badder West Side;" and after more drinking they'd lost all their caution, even -- Brandon dimly remembered -- pissing in public on wharf pilings; and he'd sprawled beside Troy on their backs in the sand, sucking down beer as fast as he could to see where it would take him.

He wondered now, here on the mattress, gazing up at the blurry light bulb, if he'd been trying to find a *time?* A better time than the one he was in... a past, future or alternate time. Smoking weed had been like that, too... at least when it was something new. Like, being stoned was only the means -- the fairy dust or clicking his heels -- to take him where he wanted to go. But he'd given up searching when drunk or high because he'd never found anything. The reason for drinking was getting drunk; the purpose of smoking was getting stoned, and there wasn't any magic gate through which to find a better time. He'd talked to Chad about that once, but his brother had only shaken his head and said it was time to grow up.

Brandon's mind returned to the present. He found he was panting for breath.

"Slow down," murmured Tommy. "You're new at this."

Dazedly, Brandon gazed around. He almost expected to see a beach, dark and deserted as night drew on. Instead, he was stuck between two sweaty boys on a mattress in Travis's tiny room, surrounded by other glistening shapes like the blubbery sea lions out on their rock. He suddenly wanted to laugh. It was funny that he could feel so good, so drunk and high, and mook-it-all free, yet not be numbing his brain with beer or dumbing it down on dope.

"It's a natural high," he panted.

Tommy grinned, his chubby face smeared with barbecue sauce. "You're getting there, Bucky."

"Then... there *is* somewhere to go?"

"Oh yeah!" laughed Zach, his chest and belly also spattered. "There's a there somewhere for sure."

"That's deep," said Brandon solemnly. "Like, today is tomorrow's yesterday."

"Hmm," said Danny, pondering. "Today was yesterday's tomorrow."

Carlos laughed. "All I know is I'm here now."

"Yeah," said Zach. "But, are you *there?*"

"I think I'm getting close," said Brandon.

"How about this one?" suggested Travis. "I know you believe you understand what you think you said, but I'm not sure you realize that what you heard was not what you meant."

"That's so cool!" sighed Brandon.

Bottles of soda were floating around, as soon as one vanished another appeared. Brandon drank deeply from each as it came. He was getting pretty sloppy about it, dribbles running down his chest,

119

slick with sweat and slathered with sauce.

"Did you ever notice," said Zach, "on the Land 'O Lakes butter box, there's a picture of an Indian girl holding a Land 'O Lakes butter box, an' on the box is a picture of an Indian girl holding a Land 'O Lakes butter box, an' on that box..."

"Deep!" sighed Brandon. "Like the meaning of life, the universe and everything."

"42," said Danny.

An infinity later in a peaceful haze, he was sprawled on his back at the edge of exploding. He hadn't found the better time yet, but this was the closest he'd ever gotten. Maybe it was an old writer's trick, but it seemed as if, *the next thing he knew*, Tommy was shaking his shoulder.

"Brandon, wake up, we gotta go home."

"Huh?" said Brandon. He blasted a burp... which felt so good he did it again. "Um, what happened?"

Tommy laughed. "Food coma."

Brandon wiped sweat from his face. "What time is it?"

"About eleven-thirty."

"We were supposed to be home by eleven!"

"Mmm?" said Carlos opening an eye. He was leaning back against the wall, his legs spread wide on the mattress. "I gotta be home by midnight." He gently jiggled his belly. "Hope I can make it three blocks."

Brandon's head lay on Kelvin's belly... rippled with muscle and tight as a drum. Someone sprawled across his legs... Ro in a slumbering mass. Zach and Danny were gone, but Travis was at his computer busily clattering keys.

"Yo, Brandon," said Travis, swinging around in the squealing chair. "You didn't say when you wanted to leave so I didn't wake you up."

"I gotta get goin'," said Carlos.

"You mean you think you can walk?" groaned Brandon. He unbuttoned his jeans, which pinched his belly, and clumsily tried to sit up. "Tommy, gimmie a hand."

Tommy laughed. "You're kidding, right?"

120

"I'm stuck," panted Brandon. "Ro's on my legs."

"I'll get him off," said Travis, dropping massively to his knees. "C'mon, little man. Time for a shower and then get to bed."

"Aight," mumbled Ro.

"Help me up, Tommy," puffed Brandon. "We don't have time for games."

"Who's playing," said Tommy. "I'm too stuffed to move."

"I know Da Beast's one weakness."

"Okay, okay!"

Ro got to his feet with Travis's help and slowly waddled into the hall. Kelvin woke up and stretched like a panther. "I give you a hand."

"Me first," said Carlos. "Hey, Travis. Tell your folks to get their joint open. I'll be their best customer. ...Bonus notches, you-all."

Tommy sighed as Carlos left. "I don't know about you, Brandon, but I'll be lucky to walk home tonight. I'm way too stuffed to skate."

"We'll take a bus," said Brandon. He burped again, then turned to Travis, who was back at his computer. "How close to midnight is it?"

"Mickey says it's 11:43."

"Are you an' Tommy in shit?" asked Kelvin.

"My 'rents won't go ballistic as long as I call before midnight. It's a deal we made last year."

Travis smiled. "Is midnight when you turn into a pumpkin?"

Brandon groaned. "My belly feels like a pumpkin! Or like I swallowed one."

"Looks like it, too," said Tommy.

"My 'rents are pretty cool," said Brandon. "Besides, I think they trust me enough to know I wouldn't get Tommy in trouble."

"Huh?" murmured Tommy.

Brandon poked him. "Don't even think about going to sleep!" He pulled his phone from a pocket. "I'll send 'em a text."

"You can take a shower if you want," said Travis.

Brandon looked down at himself, his chest and belly smeared with sauce and almost as messy as Tommy's.

"I'ma get Ro in the shower," said Kelvin. "We'll leave some hot water for you."

Tommy yawned. "Set the snooze alarm."

"Hey!" snapped Brandon. "I said stay awake! ...Listen Tommy, when we get home, you go around to the patio door and use your key to my room. I'll go in the front and take the heat."

"My hero." Tommy patted Brandon's belly. "You get some ideas about fat stuff tonight?"

"With a mookin' bullet." Brandon looked up at Travis. "Do you eat like this a lot?"

Travis laughed. "If I did I'd look like that 'toon of Ro with my belly hanging down to my feet."

"I feel like that now," sighed Tommy. "And it's bitchin' boss!"

Travis looked thoughtful. "I almost did get there." He rummaged around in the stuff on his desk and found an old Nike box. Inside was a pile of pictures. He pulled one out and tossed it to Tommy. "That's me at Ro's age."

Tommy's mouth dropped open. "COOL!"

"Woah!" said Brandon. "You were fatter than Ro is now!"

Kelvin's voice came from up the hall. "Showin' off your baby pics, cuz?"

"And that was a little too fat," said Travis.

"Mean you went on a *diet?*" asked Tommy, looking horrified.

"It's a long story," said Travis.

"Go on," said Brandon. "I have to digest before I can walk."

"Man!" said Tommy, still scoping the picture. "You musta been an immobile kid!"

"Close," said Travis. "...Well, once upon a time, there were two fat kids named Travis and Ro, who had slow metabolisms. There's a big medical word, but it basically means we were very efficient at getting fat and fatter. Like, storing up fat for famines."

"Like the Papago Indians?" asked Tommy.

"Yeah," said Travis. "But my folks didn't notice how fat I was getting."

"'Cause they seen you every day," said Tommy.

"Saw you," said Brandon.

"Nope, seen him."

122

Travis went on, "Mom and dad were working hard and coming home really tired at night. Plus, there was always Kelvin to put on my socks and tie my shoes when my belly got so huge I couldn't reach my feet anymore. I got so fat he had to help me up and down our apart-ment stairs. But I didn't care, I felt really good."

Travis glanced at the picture. "All that was all *me*. It's a powerful feeling when you're that age. To be bigger than everyone else. To make the floor shake when you walk. It was kinda like driving a bull-dozer, and I was inside controlling it. I wasn't the only fat kid in the 'hood, but I was definitely the fattest."

"Got that right!" called Kelvin's voice. "We thought he was the phattest, too."

"So did I!" called Ro. "The phattest brother in the world!"

"Anyway," said Travis. "Mom sent me down to the store one day when Kelvin was sick with the flu. *You* coulda gone there and back in five minutes, but I was gone for almost an hour. Getting downstairs was fairly easy, but waddling to the store was a struggle. And getting back up the stairs again was like climbing a mile-high mountain where every step was another cliff to get my belly over. When I finally made it to the top I laid there panting 'I did it!' like Dora. Then my mom and dad came out. They were worried 'cause I'd been gone so long. At first they thought I'd gotten jacked or beat-down on the street. But then it was like the first time they saw how fat I really was."

"Did they freak?" asked Tommy.

"Nah, they were cool. They didn't start in about diets, or act like I had a disease, but we went to a doctor next week."

"Uh-oh," said Tommy.

Travis scowled. "The doctor was white, naturally, and *he* freaked at how fat I was. Started yelling at my folks. Accused 'em of over-feeding me to keep me shut-up when I was a baby. Or neglecting me... like everyone knows black parents do."

"What an asshole!" said Brandon.

"'Specially in front of a little kid. He even threatened to call the cops and get me taken away." Travis looked thoughtful. "That was the very first time in my life when I wondered if something was wrong with me. Not only was I 'morbidly obese' ...a stupid thing to tell a kid... but I wasn't as good as everyone else."

He shrugged. "Before that happened I was just a kid who couldn't run, or walk very far, but my friends knew that. Like, physical wasn't my thing. But, I had lots of other things. I read books and rocked my grades, kicked-ass on games and drew cartoons. I started tagging T-shirts." Travis glanced around the walls at the big-eyed little chubby kids. "Those are a lot of my old designs. And friends came over to hang with me because they liked me for who I was."

"Tell me about it," said Tommy. "I have lots of things, too, but haters only see my fat."

Travis nodded. "Most fat kids have lots of things, but haters only see their fat."

"You could tag shirts at the Boardwalk," said Brandon. "Those are bitchin' 'toons."

"I might next summer," said Travis. "The guy at the shirt booth likes my work."

"What happened with the doctor?" asked Tommy.

"He finally stopped ranting how 'obese' I was and did some tests like he should have done before freaking me out and dissing my folks. He found out why I'd gotten so fat, and it wasn't from watching TV all the time, or playing games, or eating junkfood, or my folks didn't care about me. I just had a very efficient body."

Brandon smiled. "Maybe you're in the wrong time."

"I've thought that, too."

"Hey!" said Tommy. "You could have gotten in *National Enquirer*! Or on some trashy TV show. You could have made a ton of money for being the fattest kid in the world!"

"Maaaan!" said Brandon.

Travis laughed. "Kelvin had the same ideas. Like, how to turn my fat into fortune."

"Woulda worked, too," said Kelvin. He came back in all glistening black, a Beastworld prince, half panther, half boy.

"So, then what happened?" asked Tommy.

"The doctor wanted to cut me open... do that bypass thing... so I'd really never be normal, but my folks weren't having that shit. So he put me on some drugs. ...Which cost like hell, of course."

Brandon's eyes went from the photo to Travis, comparing the mammoth boy in the chair to the almost impossible younger kid whose belly hung down past his knees. "Guess they worked?"

Travis made a face. "Oh, they worked, like a cluster-bomb. ...If you don't care about collateral damage."

"Got that right," said Kelvin. "He got hyper like a crackhead an' couldn't concentrate in school."

"Or anywhere else," said Travis. "My grades went from A's to F's overnight. I couldn't even read a book. I'm never going through that shit again!"

Kelvin nodded as Ro waddled in naked and ebony clean. Kelvin ruffled the boy's locks. "An' we ain't puttin' Ro through it, neither."

Ro smiled. "Tommy's gonna teach me skating soon's I can afford a board. Skating's good exercise, huh?"

"Sure," said Tommy. "Check me out."

"Tommy's as strong as a beast," said Brandon.

Tommy laughed. "Which pisses off most of the doctors my mother takes me to."

Travis smiled. "My parents found an old-school doctor who's more concerned with how we feel instead of how much we weigh."

"He doesn't say you're too fat?" asked Brandon.

"He'd probably say *you* were too fat if you weighed as much as me or Ro. But, basically we're designed to get fat. ...And maybe we are in the wrong time."

"You don't take those drugs anymore?" asked Tommy.

"Not for years," said Travis. "I didn't *lose* a lot of weight, I just didn't gain it so fast on the drugs, so it's like I grew into my fat."

Brandon asked, "But how do you keep from getting too fat? Again, I mean? And what about Ro?"

Travis laughed and slapped his belly, making it ripple in waves. "You saying we aren't already?"

"How would I know? I'm outside, you're in."

"You are learning, Bucky," said Tommy.

"We probably are getting fatter," said Travis. He draped a huge arm over Roosevelt's shoulders. "But we're also getting taller, so maybe it balances out. But I'm down with me and I like who I am."

"Same here," said Ro, puffing his already mammoth boy-breasts until they looked like they'd fly away hissing if accidentally poked with a pin. "An' mom an' dad are down with us, too."

"Which is why you're *phat* fat dudes," said Tommy. "Hey, can I borrow this pic? I wanna make a color copy and put it up on my wall."

"Sure, man," said Travis.

"Want mine, too?" asked Ro.

"Def! And could you autograph 'em?"

"Like I'm a star?" asked Ro.

"You are to me," said Tommy. "And if you need any help with stuff, like at school or with haters and bullies, I got your back."

Brandon glanced at the monitor clock. "We better get going."

"Aight," said Travis. "See you tomorrow. ...I started on that story. The one we talked about today."

"I read a little. ...I hope that was cool?"

"What do you think?"

"It's a boss beginning. ...Is the surfer a ghost? Or did he get snatched by aliens and they brought him back in the wrong time?"

"We can talk about that," said Travis. "I was just trying to get down the scene where he wakes up on a beach in the morning, can't find his stuff but goes to school."

"Like Rip Van Winkle."

"It could work that way, too." Travis yawned and stretched. "See you tomorrow."

"Stay phat," said Tommy.

Ro slapped Tommy a five. "Phat forever, dude."

FOURTEEN

About a half an hour later, Tommy was stripped to his cutoffs again and comfortably sprawled in Brandon's chair as only a rolly fat kid could sprawl. He was scrolling the computer screen, listening to classic rock, and puffing the Cuban cigar. He also had the TV on, and Ronald McDonald was dancing around with a bunch of skinny hyper kids while singing about how healthy it was to go out and play in McDonald Land.

"How did it go with the 'rents?" he asked, as Brandon came in from the hall. "They give you the rubber hose?"

Brandon began to take off his clothes, dropping them on the floor in a trail. "Just the usual lecture about being a 'responsible teen,' but I think they were mostly relieved that I wasn't stoned again. I'm only an hour past curfew, and the reason was I hooked with some friends and we just forgot about time. No dope, no drugs, and I'm not even drunk: that makes me a DARE pledge-boy compared to the shape I was in last year."

Tommy offered the cigar. "You had me a little worried back then."

Brandon patted his bulging tummy, which brought the term, distended, to mind... he could actually feel his skin being stretched. Metaphorically with sexual shadings, it was sort of like when he'd been younger, over-indulged in jacking-off and gotten an irritated place on his enthusiastic shaft but even the pain was pleasurable so he'd kept going on. "I'm feeling really good, but I sure couldn't eat like that every day."

"Why not, if you could?"

"Well... 'cause I'd probably start getting fat."

127

"Which is totally natural."

Brandon took a puff and handed back the cigar. "A lot of things are natural, but not everybody wants to do them."

Tommy blew a smoke ring. "Such as?"

"...Well, getting older."

"You don't wanna get older?"

"Old enough for my drivers license, but after that it starts looking scary."

"Yeah," agreed Tommy. "And nobody wants to get really old. My grandfather won the battle of the bulge... the *real* battle... and now they feed him with a spoon. But, nineteen or twenty isn't *that* old, and you can drink legal at twenty-one."

"Which probably takes all the fun out of it." Brandon sat down on his bed. "I guess it's a matter of degree. Like, for a fat kid, you're just about perfect in your present form."

"Only just about?"

"Okay, to me you're the perfect fat kid."

Tommy passed the cigar. "Thanks, but why?"

"You're the one who ought to know."

"I have my reasons, but let's hear yours."

Brandon puffed smoke and studied Tommy. "You're fat enough to be fat and still be..."

"Smart, cool, and fun to be with? ...We'll also accept bitchin' and boss."

"*Déjà vu*," said Brandon.

"But I wouldn't be if I got 'obese?'"

"I don't think I'll use that word anymore, it's becoming like wop, spic and nigger."

"A lot fatter then, like Travis or Ro?"

Brandon considered. "I don't even think I'd call them too fat. They have all your bitchin' and boss qualities. ...Would you wanna get fatter?"

"My boy-breasts could be bigger," said Tommy, fondly fondling his orbs.

Brandon laughed. "Get inspired by Travis?"

"I'd cheerfully settle for Ro's. ...But, if you *had* to use the O-word, would you define it as someone too fat to be cool and fun to be with?"

Brandon considered again. "That would be like defining nigger. It's a word this society put in my head when I was to young to understand how degrading and hateful it was... a word to hate other people with and encourage others to hate... but I can choose not to use it. Or, speaking metaphorically, let myself be triggered to use it and per-petuate more hate."

"Which means you know yourself pretty well. But, you still haven't answered the question."

"The answer is 42."

"Elaborate."

"...That dude I met in P.E. today... Jason... called himself obese. He's really not *that* fat; but if I *had* to use that word I'd say it applies to him within the parameters we're discussing. But I don't think he'd be fun to be with... at least by my definition... even if he looked like Troy. ...Who seems to be *losing* those qualities in pursuit of his self-perceived perfection."

Tommy smiled. "I'd say this has been a productive session."

"Bill me tomorrow." Brandon passed back the cigar and glanced at the monitor. "Where did you go?"

"Just checking our site. A couple new posts in the guest book."

"Are they cool?"

"One of 'em is. The other one's from a retarded hater who can't even spell the O-word. ...We should do another Beastworld episode. ...Think Travis would come for a vid? And maybe Ro and Kelvin?"

"That's a boss idea," said Brandon. "They'd look bitchin' on Beast-world."

"So would Carlos and Danny."

"Have you ever asked Zach?"

"He was working all summer." Tommy shut down the computer and passed the cigar back to Brandon. Then he lost his cutoffs, climbed into bed, and sighed while gently massaging his belly. "I am soooo mookin' FAAAAAAT, and I love it!"

Brandon laughed. "Does that get you hot?"

"Watch and see. Or, better yet, participate."

129

"Would you have wanted me to, before I became fat-aware?"

"You might have gotten confused."

"Like, thought I was getting gay?"

"In your case you'd have probably thought you were taking advan-tage of me. ...Oh, by the way, I ate that Snickers bar in your desk; I'll pay you back tomorrow."

"How could you *possibly* eat something else after all we ate to-night?"

"Like you said, it's like being high and you don't wanna come down."

Brandon passed the cigar. "You always have to come down some-time. Even I figured that out. And the higher you get, the farther you fall."

"At least I'll go to sleep totally stuffed... that's another way to get fatter. And I have to put on a few more pounds so mom will see her diet's dust. Then maybe she'll leave my body alone."

"Did she ever threaten to send you to fat camp?"

"Oh sure, but I told her I'd run away."

"Would you?"

Tommy passed back the cigar. It's hypothetical, but it worked. Didn't your dad say something last year about a camp for 'troubled teens?' And didn't 'running away' come up in that conversation?"

"Yeah."

"Would you?"

Brandon took off his boxers and tossed them on the floor. "It was hypothetical, but it worked."

Tommy pointed to the TV. "There's another one of those 'eat all you want and never gain weight' pill commercials. Obviously they make you shit... yeah the possible side-effects are 'uncontrollable bowel movements' and maybe 'oily discharge.'"

Brandon laughed. "Everything comes in a pill except brains. ...That's kinda sad if you think about it. Like, it's wasting food. Like, buy and consume but end up with shit... literally and figuratively. Like, half the world is hungry, but not only are Americans getting fat-ter, we're figuring out ways to eat even more and not have to pay the price."

"What price?" asked Tommy.

"Getting fat, duh."

"That's not a price, it's a reward, like frequent flyer miles."

"But we're taught it isn't," said Brandon. "So, instead of accepting the fact that getting fat is natural, or sharing all the food we have, we flush it down the toilet. ...Or 'work it off,' or 'walk it off.' At best that's wasting food. At worst it's kind of evil."

Tommy stroked his belly. "I like to have something to show for my money. Besides, I'm surrounded by food all the time. Food takes off its clothes and jumps up an' down an' screams, EAT ME BIG BOY!"

"Shhh, the 'rents are asleep." Then Brandon smiled. "I just got an idea for a story."

"Yeah? What is it?"

"I don't wanna mook with it now. Like, it's still being born. We have to write social satire stories for writing class next week, and I just got a bitchin' concept."

He got up and flipped the cigar out though the patio door, where it hissed on the dew-sparkled grass. Then he went into the bathroom. Its opposite door swung open, displaying Chad in his birthday suit. "So, what did you get, Goldilocks?"

"Nice people knock," said Brandon.

"Since when have I ever been nice to you? Besides, you could lock the door."

"You'd think I was doing something weird."

Chad glanced into Brandon's room. "Sleeping with Tommy is weird enough, not to mention mutual masturbation."

"I seem to remember you joining us in the not so distant past, not to mention all your expert advice in expanding our self-love horizons."

Chad shrugged. "I also used to play Beastworld with you. But, like I told you today, those things are now in the past... or should be."

"That makes a sad picture," said Brandon. "Not only can't you play anymore, but you have to jack-off alone."

"I'll pretend that's profound instead of stupid and say it's called growing up. ...And, what's your penance for coming home late, now that you're more mature? ...Not."

Brandon started to brush his teeth. "I was still tried as a minor."

"When I started high school they got more strict."

"That's 'cause they love you more than me."

Chad stalked over to Brandon. "What did you do tonight anyway? Let me see your eyes! ...Okay, you're not back on pot."

"Duh."

"And you're not drunk."

"Double duh."

"And I don't see any other signs of a budding chemical romance."

"Three duhs, you're out." Brandon spit in the sink and rinsed his mouth.

"You must have done *something;* you're too happy to be organically normal."

"Let's call it just having some old-fashioned fun."

"Mom and dad bought that from you?"

"Indeed they did, incredulous one, and the truth will set you free."

"Back to square-one, what did they give you?"

Brandon racked his toothbrush. "I'm grounded the rest of this week after school. Buuuut... Are you ready for this...?"

Chad made a fist. "Are you ready for *this?*"

"I got the raise in my allowance."

"...Yeah? How much?"

"You told me not to negotiate. The big one-double-zero with all the perks. ...Does that piss you off, brother dear?"

"I know how Cain felt about Able."

"Why? We can't rewrite the past."

"No, but we can brood about it. ...Wait a minute." Chad grabbed, smelled, and licked Brandon's hand.

"Hey!" said Brandon. "That's perverted!"

"Dope doesn't come in barbecue flavor."

"Okay, Sherlock, you cracked the case. I smoked a few ribs tonight."

"Ever hear of napkins? Besides the ones you need every month?"

"Not on Beastworld." Brandon patted his jutting tummy. "If you need any more evidence..."

Chad shrugged. "Remember what I said today; that could become your permanent look. Bet you can't even suck it in."

"Should I be something I'm not for you?"

"I know everything you're not, to infinity and beyond. ...Want a ride to school tomorrow?"

"What are *you* on tonight?"

"Had a few beers. But not enough to make me like you. ...Is that a yes?"

"Actually no. My friends take public transportation."

"So, these really aren't imaginary friends made up in your lonely desperation? ...Even the kid with the tat?"

"Even the kid with the tat. Though he wasn't there tonight."

"And where was 'there,' my wayward child?"

"You mean you didn't listen when mom and dad were grilling me? That's a first for you."

"I was on the phone with Lisa. Who rates a higher priority than your post-pubescent escapades. Though I may revise the 'post.'"

"I was at the black dude's, down in The Flats."

"Hence the ribs. Elementary."

"Bite me, Chad."

"I should slap the mookin' shit out of you! ...So, let me get this straight, Goldilocks; you and Tommy were down in The Flats? After dark where the wild things are. And not only did you come home alive, but mom and dad did not produce an entire litter of screaming kitties?"

"I didn't actually say where I was, just at a friend's."

"Damn, Brandon! I wouldn't go down there at this time of night if you gave me your mookin' allowance all year! Especially now when the Boardwalk's closed and there's no easy prey for the slum-rats. The cops won't even go down there alone."

"How do you know so much about it?"

"I, too, went through a druggie phase, except I wasn't as brain-lessly blatant." Chad shook his head. "You're either the bravest twink in the world, or the absolute stupidest." He checked the clock in

Bran-don's room. "I think we'll continue this conversation at a more con-venient time. Like when I want something from you, despite you having so little to offer. ...And we're even for the scratch on the Saab."

"Okay," said Brandon. "Am I free to go?"

"Remember, big brother is watching."

FIFTEEN

The alarm clock warbled a five-minute warning, and Brandon sleepily opened his eyes. Misty gray daylight seeped in through the curtains, the sea whispered softly against the cliffs, and blackbirds chirped outside on the lawn while busily pulling up worms. He peered at the clock's ruby numbers: only 6:55. He slapped the snooze bar and muttered a curse, but then realized it was Saturday. He'd survived his first week of public school and his new friends were coming to party.

He usually woke up ready for action, and lying warmly on his belly tempted him to prolong the pleasure by making some moves on the innocent sheet, but instead he rolled onto his back and tried to recapture the dream he'd just had, of surfing a white-sanded tropical beach on a wooden antique of a long-board. Then there had been a feast by a fire and he'd stuffed himself stupid on fabulous food. The dream would have made a cool story, but like most dreams it was slipping away, and the harder he tried to recall it the faster it fled from his mind.

Mr. Akida had spoken of that, saying you had to train your brain to file away the good ideas and dig them up when needed. He'd also said writing was like body-building, something you had to do every day if you wanted to see any gain. Writing, he'd said, was actual *work*, and sometimes you didn't want to work. But, only amateurs wrote when "inspired" or waited until the mood was right. Only amateurs courted a muse; a professional author went hunting for one and brought it back alive in a cage. He'd said to imagine you had been grounded, and since you had nothing else to do, you might as well use the time to write.

135

He'd learned those things at Brandon's age while in a South African prison. His room had been a hole in the ground, and his only crime was being black in a culture that hated his color. The guards had taken his stories away and he'd had to write them all over again, resurrecting the words in his mind.

Brandon glanced around the room -- PC, TV, and stereo, DVD player, fantasy games, tons of books and magazines -- a lot of alternate choices to writing. But he'd established a nightly routine, first getting his homework out of the way then moving on to the serious stuff, the work he really wanted to do. His output had greatly increased; he was halfway through his satire story, titled *The Encourager Clowns*, and had also finished a Beastworld tale that featured Travis, Kelvin and Ro. ...They had newly escaped from the Beastmaster's lab and hooked up with Bucky and Beast.

The *Time Surfer-boy* was going well in collaboration with Travis through email and Instant Message, though Danny and Zach kept popping in with lots of friendly distractions. Brandon and Travis work-ed until ten, then went to a chatroom for fat kids and teens on one of Tommy's favorite sites. None of the dudes there were over sixteen, and Brandon was learning a lot about fat. There were quite a few mentions of food in the chats -- though that was totally normal -- but also the pressures of being fat; the constant taunting and verbal abuse that sometimes turned into fights or attacks; the insults spewed from passing cars or spit in your face on the street.

And all that hate was acceptable to people who thought they were good. There was an "obesity epidemic," and fat kids were also terrorist threats to the Great American Way.

Tommy's screen name was DaBeast, of course, and Brandon's was naturally Bucky. Travis was WoollyMammoth, and Danny was RaisedByFatWolves. Zach was GainerTeen14, and there were many other SNs that featured "belly, blubber," and "fat." A typical session went like this:

BlubberBoy: my bad self ate a whole pizza 2nite
DaBeast: only 1? not very hungry?
WoollyMammoth: i just ate my little brother

136

LardBellyKid: cool! come over and eat mine
FatYak: rents put me on weight watchers spew
Jabba: i just ate 4 of those BOK
Bucky: BOK?
Jabba: belly on keyboard ☺

The site wasn't only for gainers, and a lot of the dudes weren't trying to gain, though they liked posting pictures of their shirtless selves and being the stars of videos that featured wobbling, jiggling, bouncing, and otherwise showing off boy-breasts and bellies. Some of the dudes *were* gaining weight, but that was only natural: if you went to the beach, you came home with a tan, if you ate at McDonalds you packed on a pound.

But, getting fatter was not always caused by being lazy, too much TV, playing games, or living on-line. Most of the dudes were physically active, with lots of skaters and bicycle riders who weighed over two-hundred pounds. There was also a dude who cross-country skied (age fifteen and 250-plus), and a Cajun kid in Louisiana (thirteen and 257) who hunted and fished in the bayou. Travis was the fattest kid who'd ever appeared on the site, and Danny a very close second, but most of the dudes had tons of cool no matter how much they weighed... though Brandon suspected that Jason lurked and occasionally begged for sympathy:

Alien8ed: im obese and i hate myself!!!

Other fat kids would join the chats, usually after lurking a while to check if the site was really fat-friendly or some sort of weight-loss group in disguise. A lot of these dudes were newbie fat, as if they'd lost a war this summer and all their former friends were dead.

That was a good metaphor; a battlefield littered with fast-food remains where all the survivors were fat and lonely, wandering dazed and often confused past smoking grills and steaming deep-fryers, slogging through puddles of cooking oil, or falling into barbecue pits. The colonels and clowns who managed the war were safely entrench-ed in their corporate bunkers, frantically frying up new ammunition and couldn't be bothered with casualty counts. "Food to the front" was all that mattered, and any kid who wouldn't eat was guilty of being a traitor. Brandon had written this into his story:

"Sir! Urgent message from Jumbo Jack! The other side now has The Half-Pounder!"

"Steady, soldier! We'll counter-attack with our Three-Quarter-Pounder. And, if that's not enough... and this is classified... we're working on a One-Pounder now!"

"I've heard rumors about the Fat Boy, sir."

"It's almost ready to drop on the public. ...And, by god, if that's not enough, we'll SUPER SIZE the Big One!"

"Do you think our boys can take that much poundage... I mean, pounding, sir? Their shirts are popping buttons. Their jackets won't zip anymore. Their jeans are always slipping off. ...And the underwear situation, sir! It's reaching critical mass!"

"War is hell, soldier. But they're eating for Freedom and Happy Meals! ...Here, brace yourself with a Bucket-size Shake."

"Thank you, sir (burp), I needed that. But clothes are very important to kids. What if they had to make a choice between buying a burger or staying in style? Those baggy new clothes are expensive."

"Do you think I just fell off a hot-dog wagon?"

"No, sir!"

"We'll lick this problem, soldier! With good old American grits! ...If clothes were made a little cheaper... less material maybe. Bring back smaller sizes. Call it 'environmentally friendly'... 'saving resources' and all that bull. Keeping the world as green as a salad smothered with creamy ranch dressing. The fashion boys will noodle it out. We've all got a stake in this pie!"

"But, what if the troops won't wear smaller clothes? Especially the... er, overweight kids?"

"I don't like to hear that word, soldier. It implies there's a weight to *be* over! There aren't any 'overweight' kids in this country! They're just... Well, you're a nice husky lad. What do you call yourself?"

"...Uh, a little chubby, sir."

"'Chubby.' Now there's a tasty word. It says lovable kids and puppy-dogs. It says, hug me, you bastard, I'm cuter than hell! ...By god, that's it! Who ever heard of a bad chubby kid? ...Check the prison statistics. We'll put one in all our TV commercials. Show his tummy peeking a little... dammit he's proud to be chubby! It's the New American Way!"

"But, what about their parents, sir? We've been hearing some talk about... (gulp)... diets."

"I've had men fried for saying that word!"

"...And, the anti-obesity rants? All those public service commercials about childhood obesity being bad?"

"Soldier, I'm only going to say this once... if I could fry you for saying diet, just imagine what I'll do if you ever say the O-word again!"

"Sorry, sir."

"There's no such thing as childhood obesity! It's a lie perpetrated by skinny tree-huggers! By health-Communists and diet-Muslims! By vegetarian terrorists who'd crash a plane full of cute chubby kids into a helpless Jack In The Box!"

"...What about 'go out an play' or 'get active?'"

"That's why we have fast-food playgrounds. And don't forget who sponsors most of those children's network shows. They get a little too preachy on 'health,' and we'll hit 'em right in the breadbasket! Stuff all their 'fitness' right back down their throats till they're shitting granola and pissing skim milk! ...We'll make the chubby kid COOL, goddammit! No anti-anything campaign has ever won against cool!"

"You're right as always, sir! We'll tell kids to get active in our fast-food playgrounds."

"They'll work up healthy appetites. And our playgrounds are safer than public parks and most of the schools in America... only a few massacres now and then. We'll hire guards... at minimum wage. Make a note of that for our ghetto franchises."

"Speaking of inner-cities, sir, what if we made him a chubby brown kid? We're still taking flak about the Hispanics... never showing any, I mean."

"There's a meaty concept! And it kills two birds with one stone. ...Big juicy succulent birds. ...But, he can't be *too* brown, or the white kids won't identify with him. They're fascinated by young black males but they don't know how to deal with brown. Get one of those ambiguous types who might be anything... the beaners will think he's one of them, the wops will think he's one of theirs, and the whites will think he's a 'dude' with a tan. No accent, of course, and no ethnic crap. ...But make him COOL, goddammit!"

"In what way, sir? We can't make him smart... the Asian does that. He can't play basketball... the black one does that."

"Make him a master of video games. But not a nerd or a geek. And make damn sure they're the COOLEST games! As bloody and violent as good taste allows!"

"I'll sink my teeth in it right after lunch."

"Make it a BIG lunch, chubby! Our way of life depends on it!"

The junk-food generals should have been grateful to all the fat kids who were fighting their wars. They should have honored their blub-bery warriors for each and every pound they put on. Bellies should have been badges of glory; the bigger the better because they held more, and everyone knew that more was better and you could never have too much. Instead of ignoring their overweight heroes -- the Big Breakfast buyers, the lunch money spenders, the after-school snackers and pre-dinner stuffers -- they should have put scales in junk-food joints, and greeters with tapes to measure kids' waists. And The Chubbiest Kid Of The Day ate free! Not only free, but as much as he wanted. Even better, as much as he could! He would sit at a super-size Table Of Honor, and the menu mascot or corporate clown would stuff him into a bloated food coma.

But, why stop with chubby? If chubby was good, then fat must be better! It had to be better because it was more! Had anyone dared to think of the profits if being fat was suddenly cool? Not only would junk-food sales explode, but there would be new lines of clothing. If

140

fat was cool, then why try to hide it? Smaller and tighter to show it off; bellies half bare over low-riding jeans that weren't even meant to be buttoned. And massive new shoes to carry the weight. And tons of new comics and magazines: "The Chubby Look And How To Get It, The Blubber Belly Is In! Overhangs: How Low Can You Go? Boy-Breasts Cool, But Are Implants Safe?" ...And TV shows: "The Chubby Kids Club." ...And movie heroes: "Enter The Sumo." ...Plus stronger bikes and skateboards (Tommy was always cracking his planks).

That might be the future for American kids -- making "obesity" cool -- but Brandon's expanding knowledge of fat had revealed a darker side of the present: the "summer fat" kids were often confused, as if they'd contracted a dirty disease and everyone hated them for it. Former friends had abandoned them, often because of the rabid peer-pressure encouraged by TV and magazines, and funded by an industry making billions from diets, health clubs and pills:

"Why do you hang with that fat little pig?"

Brothers and sisters now ragged all the time: *"You're getting so fat it's disgusting! Stay in your room when my friends come over! And wear a shirt in the swimming pool, you're getting tits like a girl!"*

Formerly loving parents had turned into anti-obesity priests beating their bibles of fat-hating rants. They made every meal a torment of guilt, and every snack a deadly sin. They set weight limits and lectured on health... parroting TV, of course. They punished with doctors, diets, and fat camps, and apologized to their neighbors and friends because their kid was "obese."

And, it was always the kid's fault. If he'd been stricken with leprosy or lost a leg in an accident, they wouldn't be dissing him twenty-four-seven, or saying how embarrassed they were that he wasn't a Holly-wood boy-toy clone. But, "nobody had to be fat." It was like being a mutant kid who so-called normal people hated. Just like color or ethnicity, fat wasn't easy to hide. And it wasn't cool.

Which might have been worse than leprosy.

A lot of the kids had always been chubby – *"cute as a teddy-bear, isn't he, dear?"* -- but now they were "greedy, stupid and lazy, ugly, disgusting..." and, worse, "**OBESE!**"

All this hate and ridicule created a vicious circle... Brandon had seen it a lot this week. Fat kids stopped skating or riding their bikes; or swimming, or just going out. It wasn't because they were lazy, or actually wanted to get even fatter: instead, going out had become dangerous, like trying to live in a war zone surrounded by enemies. Being fat made you a target, acceptable prey any time, any place, for a preemptive strike on your size. There might be only verbal assaults -- *lose some weight, you fat tub of lard!* -- but attacks could also be physical – *let's beat up that obese kid, nobody's gonna help him!*

But, no matter how kids were battered, with hateful words or physical fists, the end result was the same... humiliation and constant fear. And, no place was safe for a fat kid to go; not a park or a playground, or to school or a beach. And sometimes not even a church.

Why?

Because hating fat kids was acceptable.

This, of course, completed the circle: the kids stayed home and got even fatter.

Many kids on the site had been fat all their lives, but some had never been hated before... kids who'd moved from other places where everyone accepted their size as part of being who they were. For others it seemed like an underground, a brotherhood of blubber-boys who battled the hateful health-nazis. Some had linked from "Bucky and Beast," while others had simply searched the web for references to fat.

Brandon had done several searches himself, but had found that most of the sites about fat were only commercials for losing weight, which seemed like a viral obsession. Other sites touted exercise gear, or pimped all kinds of get-skinny pills, along with a million weight-loss plans and obscenely expensive diet food. Others were hateful blogs or rants that encouraged a holy-war on fat... *If we make these fat kids miserable, then they'll want to be skinny!*

Of course, this "scared-skinny" propaganda only promoted more ignorant hate, especially from closet-haters... people who had to hate someone but had learned to shut up about blacks or gays. It sanctioned a fat-hating Ku Klux Klan that preyed on weight instead of color... a kind of health-nazi philosophy of skinny *uber alles* like Joe Slater's black-hating bible.

There was lots of fat pornography, too... make something forbidden, perverted or "dirty" and everyone wanted to see it.

There were tons of things about being fat that Brandon had never considered, like burning your belly on hot metal tables, or how to properly wash underneath if you had a huge "hanger" like Travis and Ro. Thighs that rubbed could give you a rash, but baby powder would ease it. What about getting through turnstiles? And how did you deal with safety bars on roller-coasters and theme-park rides?

Attitude counted a lot: be proud of your body and don't be a hider, show that you weren't ashamed of yourself and some of the dissing would stop. Personal mass could be a defense... fat kids were hard to shove around, and could usually shove back harder.

Brandon had met a few gainers who came to the site to brag of their weight. He still wasn't sure what to think about that, but there were other sites for them. There were also sites for immobile kids, many of whom had dropped out of school when no longer able to take the abuse. ...The vicious circle again.

Feeding was sort of like a game with invitations to meet and eat, either on cam or in person.

Admirers came in all shapes and sizes, though most were usually average kids who liked to look at fat ones. Camming and vids were the ultimate cool, fat kids proudly displaying themselves, jiggling their bellies and bobbing their breasts -- lots of Freudian symbolism -- eating, drinking or bursting their shirts while fans showered them with encouragement.

The same applied to encouragers: some were gay -- the chubby chasers -- but many more were straight. A few said they were scared of fat -- of getting fat themselves -- but wanted to feed or encourage others like getting fat vicariously.

Bloating was also a spectator sport, swilling soda or just plain water to make your belly balloon. Bloating sessions were cammed for You Tube, or often interactive.

Then there was inflation, another way to get the fat look without adding actual pounds... but also potentially dangerous.

It didn't take a psychiatrist to see that some of these kids were weird... or maybe just driven to weirdness. Or that a lot of attraction to fat was a sexual thing, as Tommy had said.

There were quite a few girls on the site, many of whom were "average" or slim, but looking for fat or chubby dudes to feed, encourage, admire, or chat. If some girls wanted muscular boys, gothic boys or skater boys, emo boys or surfer boys, then why shouldn't others want boys who were fat?

Brandon supposed that gay attractions were based on the same kinds of things.

There were straight relationships like Troy was attracted to muscular dudes. Skaters skated with other skaters, stoners stoned with stoners, gothics gothed together, and surfers surfed with surfers. So, what was strange if other boys liked other boys who were fat?

As with any website, there were many kinds of visitors, from innocent pubescent kids who only wanted friendship, to sick, perverted predators who Brandon could have shot. There were also lots of asshole haters who spewed the same old insults, plus all the usual freaks and geeks who lurked in any chat room.

Sometimes a "loser" came to the site to preach his new skinny religion, and was usually treated like one.

It really was a whole universe, and Tommy had been right to say that exploring it could take a year.

Brandon had met some fat young writers who graced their sites and blogs with stories featuring chubby heroes... kids that movies and books denied. There were also sites that featured fat art... sketches, morphs, or chubby cartoons, as well as many fat-positive blogs. The Japanese loved fat anime, maybe because of their Sumo traditions, while other people liked fat furs.

Bosco might have liked the site, but he didn't have a computer. In fact, he'd even seemed surprised that everyone else apparently did. To Brandon that was strange. It was also a little unfortunate because Bosco himself was living proof that fat kids could be cool.

Bosco probably wasn't a ghost: he'd reappeared on Tuesday morning, plopping out of the rusty van as Brandon's bus arrived. He'd been smoking a small and gnarly cigar like old Italian fishermen smoked, and was dressed in faded 501s, a Coors T-shirt, and his U.S. Keds. He still looked like a dude from the early '60s, but Brandon had never heard of a ghost who went back to his grave for a change of clothes.

Troy had made Brandon a color copy of Bosco's magazine cover - - a chubby bronze boy in ragged cutoffs, poised on a ten-foot redwood charger riding a monster indigo wave -- and the picture was taped to the wall.

Now, Brandon studied it for a moment, then parted the window curtains, seeing a typical Santa Cruz morning, everything shrouded in ghostly gray fog.

He snagged the remote and lit the TV -- Barney, retch! He made a face and surfed the channels... a commercial for breakfast at Burger King, another for Frosted Lucky Charms (they're magically spewishious), another for Malibu Barbie (batteries not included... but why did Barbie need batteries?).

There was Doctor Destructo The Planet Destroyer, Defenders of Democracy, Ronald McDonald (naturally), Frosted Flakes, Jack-In-The-Box, Taco Bell and KFC. There were commercials for Toaster Tarts, Chef Boy-ar-dee, Fruit By The Foot, and an ancient rerun of *Stop The Smoggies* with a stupid fat villain to teach little kids that nobody fat could be good.

A million channels of morning kid-shows, sponsored by junk and junkier food. Watch this, buy this, EAT THIS NOW, and if you don't you're so uncool! It was always eat or buy something -- wear it, play it, gobble it up! And too mookin' bad if you ran out of cash because Tony The Tiger would kick your ass and Ronald McDonald would spit in your face. And even worse if you got fat, because...

Because being fat "proved" you were weak?

Like kids who couldn't cope with dope without becoming addicts? That was an interesting concept; like trying to live on a planet of plenty where the meaning of life was buy and consume and still have money to buy even more.

Or, eat all the time and not get obese.

145

SIXTEEN

Brandon turned off the TV and looked out the patio doorway again: the pool lay as placid as window glass, and moisture beaded the plastic chairs, gleaming like drops of mercury, while spider webs sparkled like silvery lace.

He went to his dresser and opened a drawer. The first pair of boxers were way too tight, but they were leftover from last year. He found a recently-purchased pair, which were slightly snug when he pulled them on, and studied himself in the mirror, turning sideways and checking his tummy. He couldn't suck it totally flat, but that probably wasn't surprising... for sure he'd gained a couple of pounds after the feast at Travis's. Then there was lunch at school every day, and he'd been eating a lot with his friends, and snacking while surfing the web at home and working on Bucky And Beast. He should have expected some gain, he decided while patting his plump new prominence, though only a week seemed a little fast to build a belly he couldn't deny. ...But it wasn't his fault: if his parents hadn't grounded him, he would have been skating after school, cruising with Tommy, or down at the beach. But, he'd be skating again next week and would probably lose this extra weight.

In a way that seemed like a waste, like losing something he'd rightfully earned. He relaxed his belly and slouched, and tried to picture himself being fat. Not *that* fat, just maybe like Bosco. Or, with a basketball belly like Zach. On Tuesday, Zach's girlfriend, Nikki Barnes, had joined them for lunch in the cafeteria. Brandon had been dismayed to find that *she* was the girl in the tire-tread sandals! The girl who'd actually looked at him twice.

Brandon supposed he was envious, though he also supposed

146

that was normal. Nikki was nice, and she wasn't a tease, but he'd thought he was going to cream his jeans when she had pressed herself to Zach and lovingly cuddled and fed him.

Brandon wasn't a randy pubescent -- at least not anymore -- but he'd almost had to leave the table. He'd seen a lot more graphic displays, but Nikki had already done that to *him*... at least in his mind in the shower that morning. And now she was doing it to Zach!

Yeah, it was an ancient cliché, but he'd wondered what she could see in Zach? Like, besides a bitchin' belly, what did Zach have that Brandon didn't?

Brandon could barely swallow his fries... they could have been carrots for all he cared. The only reason he even kept eating was fear of having an "accident" as Nikki stuffed food into Zach's eager mouth. Life was so unfair sometimes. Especially when you were boringly normal.

Or maybe just boringly Brandon.

Sure, it was cool to have new friends, but it would have been cooler to have something more... like a friend with "real" breasts.

He scanned himself in the mirror again, then put on an old wife-beater. He snagged a pillow off the bed and stuffed it under the shirt. He did look kind of cool with a belly. Then he balled up boxer shorts, adding boy-breasts like Bosco's, and studied himself again. "Bucky gets fat," he murmured. "Could be the next episode."

But, it didn't look very real, even under the shirt, and Bucky didn't wear a shirt. And even Hollywood FX couldn't seem to produce realistic fat with all its rolly wobbles and wiggles, so what could he possibly make at home to fatten Bucky convincingly?

He laughed. "The real thing?"

So, what if did put on a few pounds? ...At least a few more than he already had. It would be an experiment, like research for writing a story. How would his fans react? Some would probably reject him; but would he get new ones who liked Bucky chubby?

Maybe a little reluctantly, he tossed his "belly" back on the bed and returned his "boy-breasts" to the drawer. The 'beater had stretched so he stripped it off. The air in the room felt chilly and damp. His ancient blankie, a childhood relic, lay on the foot of the bed. He draped it over his shoulders, then the phone started to ring.

"Hello?" said Brandon. "...Oh, hi, Rex. ...Nah, that's cool, I was already up. ...'Course we're still on today. I hope the mookin' fog burns off. ...Sure, come over anytime. Travis, Ro and Kelvin should be here elevenish. Danny's coming, too. So are Carlos and Bosco, but Zach has to work on the weekends as long as the Boardwalk's open. ...Yeah, I guess you would. But, not everybody needs a tan. ...Sun-screen? My mom's got some, but it smells kinda femmy. You might wanna bring your own. There's a drugstore on Mission Street before you get to Bay. ...Yeah, I wanted to score some brew, but that depends if the 'rents are here. There's a company picnic, but I'm not sure they're gonna go. ...Hey, that's cool. Like, you know what they say: 'it's okay not to drink.' ...Aight, see you later."

Brandon went to the kitchen and opened the fridge. There was stuff to make an omelet -- ham, cheese, and onion, maybe -- but Tommy would be over soon and it didn't seem right to eat without him. Brandon drank milk from the carton -- which always freaked his mom if she caught him -- then went to a cupboard for Pop Tarts and loaded a pair in the toaster.

Then he wandered up the hall, feeling alone in the big gloomy house in spite of knowing his family was there. The heating system murmured low, and yet there was still a chill in the air. He paused to peer into his father's den: its shelves were filled with classic books from a high-class book-of-the-month club. They were beautifully bound in expensive leather with gilded spines and gold-leaf titles; and though Brandon had read most of them, his dad could never find the time. The trouble with cyberspace, he'd said, was that everything moved at the speed of light and you couldn't slow down for "me time" or you'd be left behind.

The huge living room was a shadowy cavern filled with lurking furniture like creepy creatures waiting to pounce. Magazines lay on the coffee table, neatly fanned in a formal display like something in a waiting room. The Mexican maid, Olivia, arranged them when she came twice a week, though they usually didn't need it. Once, she had brought her son... maybe she couldn't find a sitter. His name was Dax and he'd been about six, as rolly as a shar-pei puppy, and Olivia

148

was proud of him. Brandon had offered to babysit and taken him out to play in the pool, where he'd disrobed to boxer shorts and floated like a happy cork.

A new thought came to Brandon's mind, one of those possible plotting mistakes that sloppy writers made. Travis had made the ghost surfer chubby -- not surprisingly like Bosco -- so how could he have drowned? ...Maybe slammed against a rock?

He opened the drapes and stood looking out. The lush lawn glittered with diamonds of dew. Pearly fog was shrouding the sea but seemed to be lifting a little. Seagulls lined the wooden rails that guarded the edge of the cliffs: they were probably also praying for sun so they could hunt for food. A jogger plodded along the path, middle-aged and that loose kind of skinny that came from losing too much weight. He wore that "running from something" expression Brandon had started to notice. A surfer rolled by on a skateboard, maybe fifteen and average build, his suit stripped down to his waist. His coppery body was glistening with fog, and his breath trailed behind like puffs of pale smoke. He carried his surfboard under an arm, and his eyes were aimed at the distant Point with its little brick lighthouse hidden in mist. Brandon remembered what Chad had said: maybe surfing *was* like a religion, and catching a wave was worshipping God?

Maybe a god from a long-ago time.

"Pray for surf," Brandon murmured.

"Brandon?"

Brandon turned from the misty scene. "Morning, mom. Did you and dad decide to go?"

Brandon's mother, Darlene Williams -- her mother had loved The Mickey Mouse Club -- was clad in a bathrobe and fuzzy slippers. She was slim and -- Brandon supposed -- attractive for an "older woman." He'd certainly gotten his share of her genes, especially her silky blond hair.

Darlene made a face. "We're going to have to, honey. I was hoping to get some rest this weekend, but ever since the Japanese buyout it's been company picnics and softball games. And you have to go or everyone talks."

"Sounds like peer-pressure," said Brandon.

"That doesn't stop when you're grown-up. ...At least you'll have the house to yourself when your new friends come over." Darlene glanced at the wall clock, a 1960s sunburst. "We'll be leaving at nine. ...You could turn up the heat if you're cold instead of wearing that ratty old blanket. Makes you look like a wild young waif."

"That's okay. The fog's burning off."

His mother seemed to hesitate. "Tommy's mother called last night. She asked if you've been... feeding him?"

Brandon shrugged. "He's my friend so we eat together. What could be more natural? And he's always had breakfast with me. Ever since we were little."

"I know, honey," said Darlene. "But his mother is very concerned. She told me he's gained five pounds this week."

"Wow, that's gotta be a record!"

"...But, honey, he's obese, and that's bad for his health."

Brandon frowned. "What about his *mental* health? From getting ragged about being 'obese?'"

"Please don't use that word, it's vulgar."

"Obese?" said Brandon. "It should be."

"I meant the other one."

"Oh. Sorry. But, she should leave his body alone and let him be who he is. Like, some kids are fat, so what? If he's happy, that should be what matters."

"But, he can't be happy being obese."

"Who says he can't be happy, mom? TV commercials and trash talk shows? Companies selling diet food? Gyms, health clubs and weight-loss groups? Intolerant ass... people, who rant everyone should be skinny? The only times he's been unhappy is when his mom is starving him."

"'Starving' is a little extreme. And he's only twelve. He's not qualified to judge how he feels. That's why children have parents." Darlene smiled. "And, he's going to start noticing girls pretty soon."

"Zot?" said Brandon.

"I have to start getting ready to go. I know you'll do the right thing for Tommy." Darlene hesitated again. "Remember when you

150

had your problem?"

"Which one? I have a huge supply."

"I don't have time to spar with you. All I meant was, you'd have had a harder time solving your problem if someone kept enabling you."

"Someone did enable me... most of my so-called 'friends' at the time. But I wouldn't call being fat a problem... though it seems to be everyone's problem who's not."

"...Well... have a good time with your new friends today." Darlene smiled. "I'd like to be here to meet them, but I guess that wouldn't be cool."

"You'll meet 'em pretty soon. This is only the first week of school."

"And you really like it there? You're not just being rebellious?"

"It has its good points."

Darlene came over, bringing the scent of sleepy woman and herbal-essence shampoo. She stroked back Brandon's hair and gently kissed his cheek. "Have a nice day, honey."

"You too, mom." Then Brandon asked as she turned to leave: "How come we stopped going to the Free Beach?"

"...Well... time, mostly. Never having enough."

"That's kinda funny," said Brandon. "Everyone wants more of everything, but the more they get the less time they have, and it's time that's really important."

"...I guess that's true," said Darlene. "But, there's less time as you get older."

"You're not old, mom." Brandon smiled again. "Remember when we played there? All of us like kids? Like, we were The Swiss Family Robinson marooned on an island all by ourselves and all we had was each other. And me and Chad were the hunter boys? ...We'd build a fire with driftwood and roast hot dogs on sticks. It was all the time we needed, huh?"

Darlene kissed Brandon's cheek again. "Thank you, honey, I needed that. Especially 'you're not old.' ...I loved the time we spent there, too. Sometimes I thought we could run away to a real island and live on a beach."

"Really?"

"Your father and I used to talk about it. ...But, everybody has dreams when they're young and think they have all the time in the world. ...Your father left your check on his desk. When I was your age you could have flown to Hawaii on that."

Brandon laughed. "Now it's a fairly cool pair of jeans."

"Levi flares were about eight dollars."

"That's an average lunch at Wendy's now. ...So, how much were islands back then?"

"Probably less than this house."

"They had some cool music back in the sixties... like *Time Has Come Today* by The Chambers Brothers."

"That was a little before my time."

"What about the Beach Boys? And The Surfaris? And Jan and Dean?"

Darlene laughed. "They were way before my time."

"Your music was mostly on records then, huh... PLs?"

"LPs. But I had eight-tracks."

"I saw one of those in an antique store. Were they any good?"

"I liked mine better than cassette, even if it did change tracks in the middle of a song. But you couldn't rewind them to play a song over. You had to let it play all the way through until it came around again."

"How come?"

"Your father explained it to me. The tape always came from the center, and you couldn't make it go backward. It always had to complete the circle and start all over again."

"Learn something new every day," said Brandon. "I hope you have a good time at the picnic." He turned back to the window.

"What are you looking at, honey?"

"The ocean. ...Isn't that why you bought this house?"

"Be sure to pull the drapes when you're through, or the sun will get in."

"You looked cool with a tan," said Brandon.

"Thank you, honey." His mom turned away. "But, sun fades the carpet."

SEVENTEEN

The shower was on his parents' bathroom, making a soothing, shivery sound, reminding Brandon of long winter nights when the ocean rushed against the cliffs and rain swished over the patio. He took his allowance check from the den, then padded into the kitchen. He pulled his Pop Tarts from the toaster, washed them down with a few gulps of milk, then went up the hall to his brother's room. He thought about knocking and hesitated, but finally just cracked the door and peeked in. Like Brandon's the place was a mess, though in a slightly more mature way probably best described as tamed. A strong scent of alcohol soured the air, and Chad lay sprawled face-down on his bed in nothing but jeans and a single sneak. Brandon approached him warily and cautiously shook his shoulder.

"Chad?" he whispered. Then louder, "Chad?"

"Uh?" Chad turned his head on the pillow.

"How was the party?"

Chad groaned. "Must have been cool, I feel like shit. ...The mook you doing in here?"

"I need a favor."

"I'd laugh except it would hurt too much. ...What time is it?"

"Mickey says seven-forty-three."

"That's obscene! Go away!"

Brandon smiled. "I know how you feel."

"I'm sure you do." Chad rolled painfully onto his back. "So, what do you want? ...Assuming I'd do something for you, which I probably won't."

"I'm having my party today..."

153

"Oh yeah, the slum-rats are coming. Be sure to hide the family jewels and put newspaper on the floor."

"Not funny, man."

Chad massaged his forehead. "Get me a beer and we *might* talk about it. ...Did mom and dad leave?"

"They're getting ready."

"Get me a beer anyway. ...And don't get caught or I'll say it's for you."

Brandon returned with a San Miguel, and Chad guzzled half the bottle. "Okay," he panted after a burp. "What do you want? ...And I'm charging you a commission."

"Not fair, man!"

"Life is so unfair sometimes, even for a privileged prince."

"Oh, give it a funeral. ...How much commission?"

"Fifty percent."

"No mookin' way! I'll shoulder-tap."

Chad drank more beer and burped again. "On Saturday morning? Good mookin' luck."

Brandon sighed. "Okay. But I'll have to cash my check."

"Sign it over to me. ...So, what do you want, Goldilocks?"

"There's gonna be nine of us..."

"Put it this way, neophyte, how mooked-up do you brats wanna get?"

"Just mooked enough to be cool. And Rex might not be drinking."

"What is he, a straight-edge? Or some kind of weird religion?"

"He's just... a little immature. In the physical sense. He's the dude who skipped a grade."

"Watch out for those geeky brainers, man. They can really kill a party. Like a skeleton at a feast. And you never know what's gonna happen if they do start drinking." Chad laughed. "Like going out with a virgin."

"Like, you're so experienced. But I think he's cool."

"Remember that when he pukes on you."

"Anyway, I want some forties."

Chad finished his beer like medicine. "Oh yeah, your new black 'homies.' Hence the ghetto theme."

"Will you shut up about that stuff? There's a brand of malt called Panther."

"Panther *piss* more like it. I tried it once, it's heinous."

"Whatever. Get ten."

"That's about thirty dollars... plus my commission."

"I can do math, boy-genius."

"So, what are your little black buds gonna eat? Fried chicken and wad-dee-melon?"

"Will you stop being a scrote! I'm getting Dominos Pizza. Plus chips and Chee-tos and stuff like that."

"At least you have good taste. Lisa had a party with 'healthy snacks' and wondered why everybody left. ...Which pretty much sucks your allowance this week."

"So now you're my financial advisor?"

"I got you that raise, didn't I? Just don't come crying to me when you're broke, I have my own expenses." Chad sat up and groaned again. "Is it hot in here?"

"No, you're just sweaty from drinking so much."

"The voice of experience. You sweat like a Turk since you switched to beer. ...And that's not a racist comment; it refers to Turkish baths."

"Duh."

Chad maneuvered his feet to the floor as if they belonged to some-body else. "Take off my shoes. ...The hell is the other one?"

Brandon laughed. "It was out on the lawn with your shirt. Don't ask me why, but I brought 'em in. And thanks for the pony ride."

"I wish you'd stop doing that to me. It's not like you're five any-more. You could break my back or rupture something. ...Take off my socks and fill up the tub."

"Hate to say it, but you really smell." Brandon glanced at Chad's weight bench. "Guess you're not gonna work-out this morning?"

Chad took several deep breaths. "Fortunately I'm in good enough shape to survive this kind of self abuse."

Brandon poked his brother's belly. "Looking a little soft right now."

"Why should I be something I'm not for you?"

"Yeah, I know your real identity."

Chad smiled. "You probably shouldn't see me like this."

"Aw, you're still my hero." Brandon knelt to untie Chad's sneak, and Chad leaned over to ruffle his hair.

"This is important, huh, twink?"

"Yeah," said Brandon. "I want a cool party."

"Don't worry, dork, I won't be here to mook with you. I'm taking Lisa to the 'Walk." Chad turned to the window. "Damn, I hope the sun comes out."

"So do I," said Brandon. "Which pretty much sucks *your* allowance, huh?"

"Hence my commission on your party pop."

"Which is obscenely extortive."

"That's the American Way. ...Help me get up."

"Wait, dammit, you're all slippery."

"Shut the mook up and take off my jeans."

"You have to let go of me first, wonder-boy. ...Put your hands on my shoulders."

"Remember, man," said Chad. "You're in control of your party, and there's no one to call if you lose it."

"Not even you? ...Where's your shorts?"

"Probably still in the tree. ...Only if your next call is gonna be to 911."

"Thanks, Chad."

"Yeah, yeah. Get me into the tub in one piece and maybe I'll drop my commission... this time."

"Wanna talk to the toilet first?"

"I should have done it out on the lawn. Just snag me another beer, I don't have time for a healthy spew. Let me sit down. Hand me my jeans." Chad pulled some pills from a pocket.

"What do those do?" asked Brandon.

"They're Lisa's diet pills. Also good for mornings like this."

"Like dexies and hydrocuts."

"Your pharmaceutical knowledge astounds me."

"Mom and dad have millions of pills."

"It's the price they pay for their success... and I'm sure you've sampled them all." Chad got up and grabbed hold of Brandon. "To the bathroom, boy, your master has spoken."

"Now I need a bath! Mook, you're sweaty!"

"It's the price I pay for my pleasure. Shut up and get me another beer."

"By the way, are they real?" asked Brandon, helping his brother into the bathroom.

"As real as Tommy's in super-size."

"So you got to second base?"

"A time to every purpose under heaven."

Tommy was at the fridge in the kitchen, gulping milk from the carton. He was barefoot and wearing an old T-shirt, but his cutoff jeans looked fairly new.

"Stealth mode," warned Brandon. "The 'rents are still here."

Tommy burped and wiped his mouth. "They give you the word... don't feed Da Beast?"

"Mom just did." Brandon snagged another beer and turned the six-pack so it still looked full.

"Isn't it kinda early?" asked Tommy. "Whew! You smell!"

"That's not me, and it's still late for Chad. I heard him come in about four. Had me a pony ride up the hall. Sometimes I actually like him. ...New cutoffs, Beast?"

"Yeah. Totally busted my old ones."

"You really gain five pounds this week?"

Tommy pulled up his shirt. "Check out that belly! How low can you go. And my boy-breasts got phatter, too."

"I'll try to resist. ...So, what's up with that? Did you decide to become a gainer?"

Tommy scowled. "This is mookin' *nuclear* war! Mom wiped my whole allowance last night! Said if I didn't lose ten pounds it was gonna stay wiped till I did!"

Brandon shook his head. "I'm more than a little confused about this."

"She's cracking, I can tell," said Tommy. "I just gotta keep the pressure on... or in my case weight. Like I said Monday night, if this diet crashes her fat war is toast and she'll finally leave my body alone and maybe admit it's mine not hers."

"But, how much fatter do you have to get?"

"Another ten pounds should prove I'm winning." Tommy guzzled the last of the milk. "What else do you have that's fattening?"

"Nothing right now till mom and dad leave. I was gonna make us an omelet."

"Make a big one. ...What's this stuff?"

"Last night's chicken parmesan. Take it in my room. ...Move your butt, here they come! And give this beer to Chad."

It was a little past nine when Brandon and Tommy returned to the kitchen. The garage door was rumbling down, and Brandon heard his dad's Explorer backing into the street. Tommy climbed on a counter stool, which took a bit of struggle. "Okay, Bucky, feed Da Beast."

Brandon took down a big copper pan from the rack over the range. "Even Da Beast might want it cooked."

"Got milk?"

"You just drank it all. And I needed some for the omelet."

"Use the quart of half-and-half, and I'll drink the rest. How about OJ?"

"In an omelet?"

"No, for me. It's fattening, too."

"Just a minute." Brandon poured two glasses of juice and handed one to Tommy.

"Pop Tarts?"

"You know where they live."

"But climbing back up here burns calories. ...Brrr! It's a little cold in here. Keeping warm burns calories, too."

Brandon glanced to the patio door, seeing nothing but grayness outside like an uncompleted universe. "I hope the mookin' sun comes out. Move over close to the stove." He turned on four of the burners, then cubed some butter to melt in the pan. "You're serious about getting fatter?"

"Ya think?" said Tommy, warming his hands at the whispering flames. "And you gotta help."

"That might not be easy," said Brandon. "Breakfast is cool 'cause the 'rents leave early. And I can feed you before they get home. And bring stuff in my room later on. But mom might wonder where all the food's going."

"Does she do a bed-check on the fridge?"

"It all goes on the computer. Like the milk you just drank." Brandon tapped keys on the Grocery Minder. "I ordered another gallon. But, what if your mom keeps calling mine and saying you're still getting fatter?"

"She can't prove you're helping me. So, how much food can you get?"

"I never thought about it. Food's just something we always have. Only alcohol needs a password. Chad cracked the code when he was thirteen, but it still shows in red. And the delivery guy has to see an I.D. We tried leaving notes... like, 'I'm in the shower'... but they're wise to that."

"We can always score beer," said Tommy. "Concentrate on food."

"But food takes up space, and mom might notice."

"What if you ordered a whole bunch of grub and stashed it in the pool-house fridge? You never use that for anything."

"It's supposed to be for party stuff, but they don't have many parties here since most of their friends are over the hill. ...Guess I could do that."

"Cool," said Tommy. "Then I can sneak over and eat it at night. If you can loan me some extra green I can eat at McDonald's, too."

"Houston, we have a problem."

"I always pay you back."

"I know," said Brandon. "But, I might not have any money this week. Thirty dollars is going for malt, and I still have to buy the party food."

"What about plastic?"

"My 'rents keep better track of theirs than your mom apparently does."

"It's the alimony and child-support. She gets way more than she spends. If dad knew how much she *doesn't* feed me, he'd take her to court for child-abuse."

"Sorry if it's uncool to ask, but you think they got divorced over you? Your dad never ragged you about your weight."

"That's one problem I don't have... blaming myself for my 'rents divorce 'cause they were fighting about my fat, but a lot of other kids do."

"It's cool you're so well-adjusted."

"It isn't easy staying that way when everyone else is going neurotic, obsessive-compulsive and schizophrenic, not to mention narcissistic, and paranoid about their weight... present company excepted."

"Thanks. But I just don't have any money to loan."

"What about your bank account?"

"I sucked it pretty dry this summer. But I'll give you my ATM card. Just don't overdraw, 'cause they let you do that so they can charge exorbitant fees."

"Thanks," said Tommy. "I'm gonna cut some lawns tomorrow. That'll help, too. Everyone loves a fat brown boy when he's working in their yard. ...Now, about those Pop Tarts?"

"You know I'm enabling you?"

"And I really appreciate it."

Chad came in wearing shaving cream. "There's some little dork at the door."

"Does he look like an elf?" asked Brandon.

"Looks like a Cub Scout selling cookies, except he's not in uniform."

"Can you put on a towel and let him in? I'm making an omelet here."

Chad came to the stove and warmed his hands. "What if I scare him away?"

"Don't tell him how dangerous you are."

"Make it bigger, I want some, too. ...And, hey, blubber-boy, I know what's up, so get off that stool and make me some coffee! I could care how fat you get, but nobody eats for free in my house."

Tommy grinned at Brandon. "Sometimes I actually like him, too."

A minute later Rex came in. He looked like he'd dressed for a surf model show in brand-new baggies and oversize tee... though all his clothes were oversize. His feet were the only big things about him, and his gigantic sneaks made a total cartoon. He wore a yellow surfer pack, along with a towel like a caped crusader, and Brandon couldn't help laughing.

"Sorry, T, but you look like an ad for Walmart."

Rex looked down at himself. "That's what you get when your mom buys clothes she thinks are cool."

"If the sun ever shines you can lose the shirt. The baggies still work. ...Oh, this is Tommy."

"Hey, Tommy," said Rex.

"Hey," said Tommy. "First party? ...Get by the fire if you're cold."

"Thanks," said Rex, coming to the stove. "First *cool* party. No ice cream and cake or stupid hats."

Tommy loaded the Mr. Coffee. "You're never too cool for ice cream and cake."

Brandon laughed. "The stupid hats come back when you're old."

"You're just in time for breakfast," said Tommy.

"I'll put some more stuff in the omelet," said Brandon. "Want some coffee, Rex?"

"Thanks, but I heard it stunts your growth." Rex pulled up his shirt, displaying his snowy white tummy. "I almost gained a pound this week."

Tommy pulled up his shirt. "I gained five."

"Woah! That's sweet! ...Can I feel your fat?"

"Sure, man."

"It's soft an' warm."

"Yeah, fat's friendly."

"I gained a little," said Brandon, turning to show off his tummy.

"Boss," said Tommy. "I'd say about three. You weigh yourself?"

"The batteries are dead on our scale."

"Cool," said Rex. "It's getting round."

"Thanks," said Brandon. "'Course, it's nothing like Tommy's or Bosco's."

"Yeah," agreed Rex. "Soft and rolly rocks. Wish I'd gained that much this week."

"I'll probably lose it again," said Brandon. "Um, do you wanna

161

get fat?"

"I wanna get big, whatever it takes."

Tommy smiled at Brandon. "Here we have a potential gainer. He has motive.... Yo, Rex, does your mom like to cook?"

"I guess so, she's a mom."

"Start telling her how good it is. And always ask for seconds. ...It is good, isn't it?"

"Most of the time," said Rex. "Except when she tries something healthy."

"No prob," said Tommy. "Start eating more of what you like and she'll probably start making more. Most moms love to see their kids eat. ...Even mine, if she'd just admit it." He turned to Brandon again. "So, besides motive, he has means as well as opportunity."

Brandon asked, "Did you ever think about working out, Rex?"

"I'd still be little, I'd just have muscles. I want mass."

"Then listen to Tommy, grasshopper."

"Aren't you gaining, too?"

"Not on purpose. I've been grounded all week and eating a lot."

"Speaking of muscles" said Tommy. "Is Troy coming to the party?"

"I asked him," said Brandon. "But he's on a diet."

"Oh my freakin' ears!"

"Said he might go surfing. Probably in Capitola down at the sewer plant."

"Did he get inspired by Bosco?"

"Maybe. ...Funny, huh? Troy inspired by a fat dude."

"Yeah, but he'd never admit it."

Brandon opened the fridge. "Want some OJ, Rex? The omelet should be done pretty soon, if I don't keep making it bigger."

"Um?" asked Rex. "Could I have a beer?"

"Change your mind about drinking?"

"Is it cool?"

"Sure," said Brandon. "My brother's gotta replace it, and we can all get primed for the party."

"Bitchin'!" said Rex. "Beer's fattening, huh?"

"It's the carbs," said Tommy. "Beer mostly goes to your belly."

Rex pulled off his shirt. "What goes up here? My chest is a joke."

"Eat a lot of starchy stuff, like mashed potatoes and Mexican food. Pasta and pizza, too. 'Course, different people get fat different ways. It depends a lot on your genes." Tommy gave Brandon a scoping. "He'd probably get baby-fat rolly like Bosco, with a cool hanger belly and bouncy boy-breasts. They're basically built the same." Tommy studied Brandon. "Even their faces would look alike if Brandon got chubby cheeks."

"Would he get innies, too?" asked Rex.

"Could happen, but they're kinda rare." Tommy wiggled out of his shirt. "Check mine."

"Cool! ...But, what do you think would happen with me? I so want a chest like yours 'cause I got nothing now."

"But you're not skinny," said Brandon.

"Just underdeveloped."

"Not for your age," said Brandon. "You're comparing yourself to older dudes."

"But that's who I'm with."

Brandon smiled. "The beasts like you for who you are, not how you look on the outside."

"I got that transfer to writing class. Now we're in four classes together."

"Cool."

"Shop class sure wasn't me! I almost got raped in the bathroom! Had to kick some dude in the balls."

"I heard shop is like practice for prison." Brandon popped the caps off three bottles. "Here, man; and sit by the fire. There's a TV if you wanna watch something."

Rex mounted a stool. "Where's the remote?"

"You have to do it manually."

Rex found the power switch. "You guys try that new triple burger at Jack's? The one they're showing now?"

"It's on my wish list," said Tommy. "After the new Taco Grande, and the super-triple at Wendys."

Rex took a sip from his bottle, then smacked his lips and drank a big gulp.

"First one?" asked Tommy. "You don't have to answer."

"First whole one." Rex drank again. "Cool house, Brandon. How many bathrooms?"

"Four. But one's for guests and we never have any."

Rex looked out through the patio doors. "Cool pool. ...Is that a sauna?"

"Yeah."

"Well, ain't this cute," said Chad, coming in. He was clad in fresh jeans and the blue denim shirt that Brandon had worn on his first day of school. "The Partridge Family's evil clones."

"You're mooking," said Brandon.

"Sorry." Chad hooked the last beer. "I'll bring your brew, then I'm outta here."

"Beer and coffee?" asked Brandon. "That's like, why bother."

"Splits the difference with Lisa's pills."

"Don't you want some of this omelet? I used all the mookin' eggs."

"Give it to Tommy, I'll dine with the King. ...Hey, Brandon, come here for a minute."

Brandon followed Chad into the garage. "How old is that kid?" asked Chad.

"I told you, thirteen."

"Well, he looks eleven. And I guess he changed his mind about drinking?"

"Obviously," said Brandon. "But Travis's little brother drinks beer, and he's really only eleven."

"But you said he was fat, and mass does matter with alcohol." Chad glanced into the kitchen. "That little twink is gonna be mooked on half a forty or less; and if something serious happens to him his 'rents might try to blame it on you."

"Are you saying I shouldn't let him drink when everyone else is gonna be? That would really make him feel little."

"I'm warning you to watch him, that's all. And call me if you start losing control. Or even if you think you are. ...And, nobody else gets into this house except the dudes you invited." Chad smiled. "I trust you more than you think I do. I just don't want the crib shot up. Or

164

you, either, Goldilocks."

"Thanks, Chad. But, won't it piss you off if I call?"

"Sure. But it's an excuse to slap you around. Not that I need one."

"You're boss, big bro."

Chad ruffled Brandon's hair. "My baby-brother's first real party. Seems like only yesterday you were learning how to tickle your Elmo. My, how time does fly."

EIGHTEEN

"**B**oss party, Brandon!"

Brandon smiled. "Thanks, T."

They stood in the kitchen doorway surveying the scene in the sun-sparkled pool. The dudes were playing water hoops, and waves were slapping the turquoise tiles like surf across the patio. Brandon's bedroom door was open, and rock punched the air from his stereo. Bowls of Chee-tos and chips stood on tables, while forty-ounce bottles were scattered around within easy reach of the boys in the pool... Travis, Carlos, Danny and Ro. The fat boys floated effort-lessly, while Kelvin had to paddle or sink.

Brandon glanced at the kitchen clock: the time was almost noon. The other dudes had arrived at eleven but Bosco still hadn't shown. Maybe the surf had been too tempting and Bosco had gone to worship his god?

As Chad had wisely predicted, Rex was mooked on the one San Miguel and just about half of a forty. He leaned against Brandon, a drunk little elf, his oversize baggies at maximum sag and slipping ever lower. "Can you put shum... some sun-screen on my back? I burn real easy."

"Sure, man," said Brandon. "Where is it?"

"In my pack... shum... somewheres."

"It's over there. C'mon."

"This is so cool!" giggled Rex, swaying a bit on his big puppy feet as Brandon rubbed the stuff on his back. "An' don't forget my butt if it's showin'."

Brandon laughed. "Lose your baggies if you want; everyone else is natural out there. That's why my 'rents had the fence put up."

166

"How come you're still wearin' jeans?"

"I have to answer the door if Bosco ever comes. And the pizza's on its way."

"I gots a small butt." Rex burst into laughter like drunk kids did. "I gots a small ever-thing!" He jerked the knot on his sagging shorts and let them drop to the floor.

Brandon smiled "Like you said, you're normal little. Wait till you grow into those feet. You know what they say about having big feet."

Rex giggled again. "Oh yeah." He hefted his forty with both little hands and took a beast-size gulp. Dribbles ran sloppily down his chin, and he came up for air panting hard. "Now do my chest... Ha!... If you can find it! ...Do me the mook all over, man! I can't even find my shelf... self anymore."

"You better do your own special place. For obvious reasons."

"...Huh?" Rex looked down, almost losing his balance. "Woah, Brandon! I didn't know!"

"You're cool, it happens to me all the time."

"But, I can't go out there like this."

Brandon rubbed sunscreen on Rex's chest. "Think about something you really hate."

"I really hate my little body."

"There's nothing wrong with who you are, and who you are is who we like."

"Check my belly, it's sch-tickin' way out!"

"Brew does that."

"Bitchin', man! I want a lot more!" Rex gulped from the bottle, leaning way back. He lost his balance and Brandon caught him.

The doorbell rang. "Hope that's Bosco," said Brandon, returning Rex to an upright position. "You're all greased up, so go be a beast."

"But, what about this?" asked Rex, pointing down.

"Think about homework."

"Nah, I'll think about bein' little."

Brandon checked the door monitor. He wasn't worried about getting banged, though a neighbor might have called the cops to investigate his colorful guests. But it was Bosco out on the porch, and the rusty old van was parked at the curb, the ancient red long-board strapped to its roof.

Bosco wore only his ragged cutoffs, plus the little tiki god between the bobby spheres of his chest. He was puffing a pungent little cigar and blatantly toting a case of Bud, though it hadn't been BYOB.

"Hi, Brandy-buck," he said as Brandon opened the door. "Sorry I'm late. I overslept. Friday night, heh, you know how that is."

"That's cool," said Brandon. "You're here now." He glanced at the van. "Who drove you?"

"I come with my Big Kahuna but I dropped him off at the Point. Give him a board an' a sixer or three an' he's totally heilotropic. ...Is my 'dub okay where she is?"

"It's only two-hour parking unless you have a permit."

Bosco gave Brandon the beer. "I'll put her in your driveway, but I might need a push to start her."

"I know it isn't far from the Point, but aren't you taking a chance by driving?"

"I gots a license."

"Zot? ...Excuse me for asking, but how old are you?"

"Fourteen, I guess."

"...You don't know?"

"Does anybody really know? It's just what people tell ya."

"...I never thought about that. So, how did you get a license?"

"In Hawaii. It's agroculturic."

"Zot?"

"Like, for kids who drive pineapple trucks."

"That's really boss! ...But is it legal in California?"

"Guess I'll find out if a cop ever stops me."

Brandon hadn't had many parties, and most of them had been ice cream and cake, but this was the best party ever! Nobody got totally mooked, except Rex, who passed-out in a patio chair; and Kelvin had lain him on Brandon's bed so he wouldn't go toast in the sun. Chad phoned in about every hour to see who'd gotten shot or stabbed, but so far the death-count was zero.

Brandon showed Bosco his surfboard, which hadn't come down from the rafters yet, and suddenly there were surfing lessons going on in the pool. Bosco toted in "Big Bertha Red," his own trusty steed from the roof of the van; and even Travis was up like magic while everyone else made waves for him. Tommy and Ro put on their cutoffs and went out front with Brandon's skate. Then everyone else came out to watch, gathering in the open garage. Ro was skating pretty well considering his awesome weight, except for always losing his jeans.

Travis laughed, watching his brother land on his butt, which look-ed like an earthquake in ebony Jell-O. "Just getting up is good exercise when you weigh as much as him."

"Wanna check it out?" asked Brandon.

"I'm way too fat to skate."

"Just get on deck and I'll push you."

"Think your board can take me?"

"Only one way to find out."

"Boss board, Brandy," said Bosco, admiring Brandon's skate. "I like them gnarly curves."

"Thanks," said Brandon. "What kind do you have?"

"Just the regular kind. She's in my 'dub."

"That's *your* ride?" asked Carlos, clad in a pair of sagging shorts and holding a bottle of Bud.

"Bought her on Molokai this summer, back when I still had some moola."

"From winning the surfing contest?" asked Brandon.

"Yeah, but I can't remember where most of the money went." Bosco patted his belly and laughed. "But a lot of it went in here."

"You never got any modeling jobs?"

"Nah."

Danny Little-Wing, a mammoth mass of burnished copper spilling over his cutoff jeans, took a swallow of beer and burped. "What about ads and movie offers?"

"Nah," said Bosco. "They gave all them goodies to the dude who won Second. He looked a lot like Brandy."

"That sucks, man," said Carlos.

"It's size discrimination!" snapped Tommy.

Bosco smiled. "I'm the star of my own life, dude. Why would I

169

wanna be anyone else's?"

Everyone followed him to the van. "Check it out," said Kelvin. "It's got an eight-track player!"

"My dad's got one," said Travis. "He still has a lot of old black tapes from the 1960s."

"They got eight-tracks now?" asked Bosco.

"Huh?" said Brandon, and studied the player. "What's that?"

"Just a regular four-track. I got mostly surfin' tunes. Want me to put somethin' on?"

"Sure," said Brandon, scanning around the van's interior and noting another tiki god hanging from the rearview mirror.

"Gotta turn on the converter," said Bosco, flipping a switch on the dashboard. "Six to twelve volts." He popped a cartridge into the player and *Surfin' U.S.A.* by the Beach Boys echoed from a small set of speakers.

Brandon somehow wasn't surprised when Bosco produced a plain wooden plank about two feet long by eight inches wide and painted bright red like his surfboard. Its wheels were made of... steel.

"That's a mookin' classic!" said Tommy. "It's gotta be sixty years old!"

"Nah," said Bosco. "Built her in June."

"Zot?" said Tommy.

Bosco decked and rolled away, cutting gracefully down the drive. The rattle of steel across cement was a strangely haunting sound, though Brandon had never heard it before. Bosco burned past Tommy's house, cut across the street and along the cliffs, then came rocketing back.

Brandon felt a strange sensation, almost like a vision: there was a chubby boy in cutoffs, shaggy-haired, tanned to the max, and riding a piece of wood on wheels. What a bitchin' concept!"

"He can't do that!" blurted Tommy.

Brandon blinked. Bosco was rolling up the driveway, past the battered safari van, while surf music twanged in the summery air. The sparkling ocean lay at his back, and there in the distance were boys on boards. What had it been like in that time?

Travis was also surveying the scene. "Not so boss for us."

"Did I say that out loud?" said Brandon. "I thought I just thought it."

"Whatever you did, I heard it." Travis looked thoughtful. "Ever feel like you were somewhere before?"

"You mean *déjà vu*? A few times."

"*You* might have been in this picture before, but when could I have been in it?" Travis scoped around again. "So, why did I feel like I was for a second?"

"Black kids must have surfed and rode skateboards in the 1960s," said Brandon.

"If they did, I never heard of it. From what I've read, we started out riding the ass-ends of busses and finished up with the Panthers. We had something to accomplish. We didn't have time for surfing and skating."

"But maybe you did... somewhere?" said Brandon. "Like, maybe you did accomplish your mission? ...Or, maybe you didn't have to?"

"You're suggesting a parallel universe? The same but not exactly the same as the one we're in here?" Travis scanned the sunlit scene. "Like, maybe in 1963... the alternate 1963... America gave us our Civil Rights? Rights we should have had all the time. And there wasn't a Vietnam War starting up. No beatniks morphing into hippies to grow their hair long and fight the System."

"Yeah," said Brandon. "Like, maybe what should have been really was in that alternate universe."

"And all this kept going on?" said Travis. "Skating and surfing, beach parties and beer?"

"Like *Endless Summer* for real," said Brandon. "But, now... or then... it was everyone's summer. Like it should have been all the time."

Travis's face grew thoughtful again. "My grandfather had to fight in that war. Then for his rights when he got home. He said it changed a lot of things, and lots of them weren't good. We got our rights on paper but not in realtime. A lot of the Panthers were murdered by the FBI. Then drugs started flooding the inner-cities. Most of the hippies cut their hair and traded love and peace for money. And the war went on for a lot more years."

171

"I've read about that," said Brandon. "This country was having a war with itself... equality versus discrimination. Love and peace against hate and war. Hawks against doves, straights against hippies... straight meant something else back then."

"Pardon me, but that's a duh."

Brandon went on, "There's a theory... time can split if it gets too stressed. Like, pulling paper until it tears."

"I've read that, too," said Travis. "Part of time goes one way, and another part goes another way."

Brandon nodded. "Usually there's only one future, and that's determined by the past. It's called the most likely future, based on where the past was headed and what would be most likely to happen if it kept going that way. ...Like, walk down a muddy road and you'll probably get muddy."

"Yeah," said Travis. "But sometimes there's a fork in the road. And time can't decide which one to take, so it splits and two futures happen."

"So, maybe that really happened," said Brandon. "Like, somewhere in the 1960s. Surf music ruled in '63, but then there was the British invasion, the Beatles and the Rolling Stones. It was like there was suddenly two kinds of rock and kids had to choose which one to follow, so suddenly there were two kinds of kids. It was also how they wore their hair, and the way they dressed. Most kids basically dressed the same until the early '60s... like in *Leave It To Beaver*... but then that suddenly changed, and how you dressed became who you were, just like the music you listened to."

Travis nodded. "Same with the split over Civil Rights. And, to be for or against the war. All that would have really stressed time."

"So, maybe time did split?" said Brandon. "And instead of one future, there were two."

"So, which was better? ...Or is better?"

Brandon glanced at Bosco. "Judging from our present... the world full of wars, school massacres, and people hating everything from skinny jeans to super-size kids... I'd say the answer was obvious: the present future from Bosco's past. *We're* in the future that took the wrong road between *Leave It To Beaver* and the Kent

State killings."

"Between Kennedy and Nixon, according to my grandfather," said Travis. "America started the 1960s going to the moon, but ended up in a war it would lose while people were fighting each other at home." Again he studied the sunlit scene. "Too bad we can't jump to Bosco's present; his future got the best of the past."

"Yeah," agreed Brandon. "And he brought some of it with him today. Like a beach party for everyone, no matter what color, shape or size. ...But you don't *really* think...?"

Travis smiled. "The answer is 42."

"Deep story, huh?"

"And it's gonna get us an A."

Brandon sighed. "I used to try to get 'here' on weed. I didn't know where I was trying to go, but maybe it was the other future and there was a way to jump across. I always had a feeling there must be somewhere better than now."

"I think everyone has that feeling sometime, but most people learn to ignore it," said Travis.

Brandon shrugged. "Maybe it's called growing up."

"He can't do that," said Tommy again.

The scene might have shifted again, just a bit, like something caught in an eye-corner glance or seen though a shimmer of heat. Again, Brandon blinked. For just a second he could have sworn that the cars driving past were bigger and older... very big and very old like the classic cars at The Beach Street Revival. And a chubby black boy in nothing but jeans was riding by on a Sting Ray bike, like one he'd seen in an antique shop.

Then all the cars were small again, and a skinny white kid rode a BMX.

"What can't Bosco do?" asked Danny.

Tommy was looking confused. "What he did over there on the edge of the cliffs. ...Didn't you see him jump over the rail? ...And then jump back again?"

"He just did an ollie," said Carlos.

"But there's *nothing* on the other side! Nothing but air and ocean!"

Danny laughed. "Maybe you've had enough brew for today?"

Sparks flew bright from Bosco's wheels as he skidded his board to a stop.

"How did you do that?" Tommy demanded.

"Do what, dude?" asked Bosco.

"Your board's got no tail so how can you jump? And even if you could have jumped, you would have gone over the cliff!"

"I didn't see him jump," said Brandon.

Tommy almost howled, "He did!"

"Maybe Danny's right?" laughed Ro, balancing on Tommy's board, his belly swinging side-to-side like a massive ebony pendulum. "You're just a little slammed."

Tommy looked about to explode. "I know what I mookin' saw, dammit!"

Travis turned to Bosco. "Did you jump over that rail?"

Bosco shrugged, "I was just enjoyin' the ride, goin' where it took me."

"It took you over the cliff!" cried Tommy.

Brandon laughed. "Slow down, Beast."

Tommy took a swig from his bottle. "I'm not new at this!"

Bosco wiped sweat from his face and laughed. "It's time for a beer."

The boys messed around with the boards for a while, Bosco checking out Brandon's plank -- though not busting any impossible moves -- while Brandon tried out Bosco's. Brandon found that Bosco's board was like learning to skate all over again. Or maybe for the very first time. Steel wheels on pavement were treacherous, skidding unexpectedly; a piece of gravel was instant doom, and none of his moves or tricks would work. It was like trying to fly a tank.

"Never done that," said Bosco, after Brandon managed a ghost of an ollie that felt like the first in history.

"Yeah you did," said Tommy. "And a lot better than Brandon."

Brandon shook his head. "Nobody could get much air on this."

"I'll put a tail on the next one," said Bosco.

Travis chuckled. "Maybe you already did."

NINETEEN

The present was past before Brandon knew it.

"Brandon!"

Brandon seemed to wake from a dream. The sky was dimming to purple and rose, and shadows were stretching out long and thin. The music had died a long time ago but no one had bothered to change the disk. Brandon sat on the edge of the pool sharing one of Bosco's cigars, his legs in the gently lapping water. Kelvin drifted asleep on the lounge, and Travis lay in the shallow end, his massive belly half afloat, his head pillowed on his arms on the steps, while Ro and Tommy dozed on the surfboards. It was like an imagined scene on Beastworld, though Carlos and Danny had said goodbye and left a little while ago.

"Your Big Kahuna?" asked Bosco, sitting next to Brandon, their shoulders occasionally touching when passing the cigar.

"Looks like I'm busted," said Brandon, glancing around at the empty brew bottles, of which there seemed an amazing abundance as if double the number of people had partied.

Tommy stretched and yawned. "Do you care?"

"No way, man, they can kill me now. Except for real sex I've had a good life, and I feel like I lived the best part today."

Travis chuckled. "It's been boss."

"And bitchin'," said Ro.

Brandon got up and shook back his hair, then went to where his father was standing just inside the kitchen doorway. His mother was hovering back by the range, and they hadn't turned on the lights. His father, Trent, was a good-looking man with just the hint of a belly bulge beneath his company T-shirt. He'd started dyeing his hair this summer... something about maintaining an image. He'd gotten a little sunburned today, though now his lips were nearly white.

"What... in... hell," he practically hissed, "do you think you're doing, young man?"

"That's a dead cliché," said Brandon.

Trent's eyes flicked to the pool, but seemed to shy away for some reason. "Look, Brandon," he said, keeping his voice under low control. "I can see what condition you're in, and it's not the time to engage, but this is just a little *too* much. Even for you."

"It's public school," said his mother. "I knew it was going to be a mistake. Just like it was for Chad."

"Don't even go there!" snapped Brandon.

His father scowled. "This isn't the time for that discussion." He turned to Brandon again. "I might excuse the drinking, but..."

"Zot?" Brandon's eyebrows went up. "But, what?" He turned to look at the other boys, who were casually donning their cutoffs and shorts.

His mother spoke from back by the stove. "Is that why you asked about the Free Beach this morning? Were you seeking confirmation?"

"Zot?" said Brandon again. "...No! I thought it was cool, that's all. ...Am I missing something here?"

"Am I missing something here?" asked Chad, coming in from the hall in just sandy swim trunks.

"Chad..." said Trent in warning.

"Who's old vee-dub safari is that? I can't get my car in the driveway."

"Chad!" snapped Trent. "This is a lot more serious than parking your goddamn car!"

"You manage to mook it up, Brandon?" asked Chad.

"Shut up, Chad!" yelled Trent.

Brandon demanded, "What are you talking about, dad?" He turned to his mother. "I thought it was cool."

"You said that already," said Chad.

"Chad, shut up!" roared Trent.

"It *was* cool, Brandon," said Darlene. "But, not in mixed company, honey."

176

"Not here, anyway," said Trent. "There are times and places for... things like that. And this isn't the time and place for... this."

"What the mook?" yelled Brandon.

"Please don't use that word," said Darlene. "It's just like saying the other one."

"Hmm," said Chad, coming to the door. "What 'mixed company' do we have out here? Are you talking about the races?"

"Chad!" yelled Trent.

"Shut up, right?"

"I think you'd better go to your room."

"I never thought you were prejudiced, dad. Or don't you like fat kids? ...And, man are they ever!"

"SHUT UP, CHAD!" bawled Brandon.

"I'm *not* prejudiced!" bellowed Trent. "...And what the hell are you talking about?"

Chad broke out laughing. "They're *boys*, dad." He patted his pecs. "Though it's understandable why you might have thought otherwise."

Trent's face flashed as red as a stoplight. Brandon's mother came to the doorway. "They're just so... dark."

"So fat, too," said Chad.

"Shut up, Chad!" yelled Brandon.

Chad grinned. "Any more weighty problems, just call me. Guess I'll be in my room."

Trent frowned. "We may have other things to discuss. ...Such as enabling your brother."

"I don't know what you're talking about, but keep your sense of humor. It's a proven survival factor." Chad went back up the hall.

Trent faced Brandon again. "I'm sorry for the... misunderstanding. It's been a long day."

"Did you have to play ball?" asked Brandon.

"Don't try to distract me." Trent seemed to study Travis and Ro as if to confirm what Chad had said. "I know we never discussed any rules about you having parties..."

"Maybe because I've never had any except for ice cream and cake."

"But Chad has. And he should have passed the rules on to you." Trent turned to Darlene, who was still gazing out at the boys. "Is there anything you'd like to say?"

"There ought to be help for children like that. They're so obese."

"Mom!" yelped Brandon.

"I'm talking about our child," said Trent. "And obesity isn't one of his problems."

"Well... assuming we're being adult about this, I'd say he has a good defense. At least on the technically that nothing was expressly forbidden." Darlene turned to Brandon. "Though your drinking worries me. Almost as much as the drugs."

"You're not back on drugs?" asked Trent.

"Nope," said Brandon.

Trent considered. "I'm assuming there hasn't been any trouble? I'm not going to hear complaints from the neighbors? Or the police?"

"Nope. *Nada*. Zip. Zilch."

"Don't be smug, Brandon, you haven't won anything."

"It was a bitchin' party, dad."

"...Well..." Trent turned to Darlene. "As long as there hasn't been any trouble."

Darlene touched Brandon's shoulder. "You know you don't have to drink to have fun?"

"Yeah, but this was the right time."

Trent smiled a little. "You seem to have acted responsibly... at least considering. Your mother and I will go have some dinner." He glanced at his Seiko. "Shall we say about an hour?"

"Sure, dad. And thanks."

Darlene smiled. "Acquitted, Brandon, but not innocent."

"Thanks, mom."

His parents left. Travis came waddling up to the door along with Roosevelt. "Brandon lives," said Travis. Ro giggled.

"What was the problem?" asked Bosco, ambling over, cigar in hand.

"Mistaken identity."

"Do we look like somebody else?" asked Kelvin.

"Nah, man. It's cool."

Tommy came up. "You gonna get grounded some more?"

"I don't think so. They gave me an hour to clean things up."

"Aight," said Ro. "Let's get busy."

About fifteen minutes later, the bottles were in the recycle bin and the bowls were stacked in the dishwasher. Bosco sauntered into the kitchen toting Big Bertha Red.

"Boss party, Brandy! Let's do it again some time. An', we'll finish them surfin' lessons out in the ocean next week. ...Any you dudes need a ride somewhere?"

"Yeah," said Ro. "Down to The Flats."

"C'mon, dudes. See ya, Brandy."

Brandon and Tommy came out to watch as the other boys piled into the van, Kelvin helping Travis and Ro climb in through the double doors on the side, which flattened the tires noticeably, while Bosco tied his board on the roof.

Brandon patted Tommy's belly. "Get more ammunition to fight your war?"

"There's still some pizza left, I'll add it to my arsenal."

"They need a push," said Brandon. "Or will that burn off your valuable fat?"

"Da Beast always up for a noble cause no matter what da sacrifice."

A few minutes later they stood on the sidewalk, watching the van's little ruby tail lights dwindle away down the street. The twanging beat of *Surfin' Sarfari* echoed over the quiet sea, which glimmered beneath the silver stars. The lighthouse flashed its beam on the Point; dew glittered like jewels on the neighborhood lawns; and a sea lion sleepily barked in the distance.

Brandon sighed as the van disappeared. "It's kinda like saying goodbye to the summer. Like, Bosco took it with him."

"Why not, I think he brought it," said Tommy. "Like you were talking to Travis about, he's got the summer that should have happened right there in his van... sorta like a Tardis."

Brandon glanced across the street to the placid ocean beyond the cliffs. "What was that stuff about him jumping?"

"Swear to god I seen him do it."

"Saw him do it."

"Espied him do it." Tommy shrugged. "But maybe the sun was in my eyes... for lack of a logical explanation."

Chad came out of the house, still in sandy swimwear and smoking a Cuban cigar. "Houston, you have a problem."

"Zot?" said Brandon.

"A responsible host always counts his guests. Some check in, but they don't check out. ...Like that little bare babe on your bed. Who mom and dad fortunately didn't see, or you wouldn't have gotten off so easy."

"...Oh shit!" said Brandon. "Rex was supposed to call his mom to come pick him up!"

Chad flicked ashes from his cigar. "Lucky for you he's still alive. *Never* leave a drunk kid on his back! If he puked, he could suffocate!"

"Did you try to wake him up?"

"I rolled him over and checked his pulse, but I don't think he'll be leaving tonight. At least not under his own power." Chad blew out smoke. "Would you care for an expert opinion?"

"C'mon, Chad! This is serious!"

"Don't panic, you're still in control... though it's slipping. Plan A: call his mom and hope she'll let him sleep over. Like, he's having so much fun here. And he thought if *you* asked...? And sound real nice; moms like nice kids to like their kids."

"...Okay," said Brandon. "But what if she won't let him?"

"Plan B: you can try a cold shower and coffee, but give yourself plenty of time. He'll still be a drunk little kid, but his mom might accept that as part his passage to getting all growed up."

"What about Lisa's diet pills?"

"Do you *want* to kill him?"

"'Course not!"

"Then I don't recommend Plan C of chemical reanimation, considering his lack of mass. ...Back to Plan B if you have to use it, and his mom freaks 'cause her baby got mooked: your ass is still pretty well covered in the legal department as long as you can establish: A, he knew before he came that there was gonna be drinking, and, B,

180

nobody pressured him to drink."

"That's kinda cold," said Brandon.

"As you sail the stormy sea of life, you might have to toss a few friends to the sharks to keep your own little boat afloat."

"Have you?"

"Thus far no. But, spit-and-shake-hands-swear-to-god loyalty is sadly a thing of the distant past, when boys had only one pair of sneaks and packed slingshots instead of AKs." Then Chad cocked his head. "And, why are all your new friends fat?"

"Like Rex and Kelvin?" asked Tommy.

"Stay out of this, fatso."

"They're not all fat," said Brandon. "Unless you spell it with a P."

"I'll rephrase the question: why are none of them normal?"

"You saying Kelvin's not normal?"

"Don't pull the race card," said Chad. "I'm prejudiced for practical reasons but I don't have a sheet in my closet."

"Bosco has a drivers license."

"...That's definitely phat with a P. But also not very normal."

"And my private school druggie friends were?"

"At least they looked normal in this neighborhood. ...Didn't you see all the curtains flutter when your new 'posse' rolled away?" Then Chad laughed and dug in a pocket. "Here's what's left of your allowance. About enough for a Happy Meal, as long as you don't want it super-sized. ...So, was being 'phat' for a few hours worth it?"

Brandon's eyes drifted back to the lighthouse flashing its beam on the starlit sea. "Yeah."

TWENTY

"Studies have shown," said the teacher, reading from a textbook, "that obese children become obese teens more frequently than normal children."

Danny Little-Wing murmured, "Just can't get away from the O-word these days."

Travis nodded. "And note the implication that fat kids can't be normal."

"...Other studies," the teacher read on, "have shown that obese teenagers are likely to become obese adults."

Kelvin yawned. "Obese sounds worse than just bein' fat."

Brandon added, "And anyone who doesn't agree is probably 'aiding terrorism' instead of thinking for themselves."

Travis said, "Most anti-obesity propaganda is based on junk science studies... propping up a premise that people have been taught is true but was never objectively proven."

"Yeah," agreed Brandon. "Once something is supposedly proven, other people 'prove' it again without doing any more research or checking any other things that might have led to a false conclusion. ...Like, 'black people tend to be violent.'"

"Don't forget brown people, man," said Carlos.

"Yeah," said Rex. "But when they want to 'prove' something, they ignore all the other possible factors that might have led to a false conclusion."

"Like comin' up poor in the 'hood," said Kelvin.

"Right," said Danny Little-Wing. "They want to 'prove' being fat is unhealthy, so they only use data that seems to prove it."

"Yeah," said Zach. "Like, those anti-smoking ads sayin' second-hand smoke gives kids asthma... they ignore all the air-pollution from factories an' power plants, an' all the exhaust from ten-billion cars. Everybody smoked when my grandma was young an' she never met a kid with asthma, but now when a lot less people smoke a lot more kids have asthma, but they try to blame it on smokers."

Carlos nodded. "If they can't make people stop doin' somethin', they try to prove it hurts other people."

"Basic peer pressure," said Brandon. "Johnny threw a spitwad, so the whole class has to stay in from recess. Which 'proves' that throwing spitwads is bad for everybody."

"Yeah," said Rex. "An' they beat the shit out of Johnny instead of thinkin' they got a bad teacher."

"An' hate-on smokers," said Zach, "instead of tryin' to stop real pollution."

Travis nodded. "Now they're trying to 'prove' that being fat hurts everybody, so everybody should hate fat kids."

The teacher droned on in a tedious voice that could have put a meth addict to sleep: "There are many serious health risks associated with being obese, and it has also been proven that obesity is harmful to society as a whole."

"I rest my case," said Travis.

The teacher was Mr. Mortimer, a pale and cadaverous-looking man who might have been in his middle forties, though usually acted twice that age and walked with an elderly stoop. He never taught if he could recite, or better yet read from a book, and he taught what passed for Health and Science... at least in public school. But, most of the students weren't listening to all the evils of being obese: the class was right after lunch, and most of the kids were sleepily stuffed.

Brandon's eyes were lured out the windows to a sunlit setting of leafy green. Trees and bushes bordered the school and seemed designed to distract a mind on a drowsy afternoon like this. It had rained a little on Thursday night, but had cleared again by morning, and the weekend weather was going to be good. Perfect for surf, according to Bosco.

The "beasts" all sat in the rear of the room. Brandon had started calling them that, and the tag was going viral. A senior had said it in

P.E. today -- assuming he'd found a new hate-word -- and the Pig-Pen had suddenly been renamed, referred to now as Beastworld.

In the last row of desks were Brandon and Rex, Kelvin, Travis, and Bosco. Danny, Zach and Carlos were in the next row up. Jason also had this class, but always sat at the front of the room and seemed to be paying the most attention to why he should hate being fat. Bosco had fallen asleep at his desk, his hair completely hiding his eyes.

Zach was nearly asleep because he'd eaten a ton at lunch. But instead of Nikki feeding him, they'd invited Brandon to do it. They had taken their food to Homicide Hill -- named for a "tragic incident" -- which overlooked the parking lot in the shade of a mammoth oak tree. There were condoms and cigarette butts in the weeds, broken crack pipes, a tampon or two, even an old hypodermic syringe; and being caught there meant instant suspension.

It had probably looked ridiculous, Brandon force-feeding shirtless Zach and stroking his bulging red-striped belly, which looked about ready to pop, under the eyes of cynical squirrels who'd probably witnessed everything from sweaty teen sex to a gang massacre, while Nikki urged them on; and he didn't need Tommy's counseling to get the Freudian symbolism with Zach's shaft straining the fly of his jeans as if to burst out like The Alien's baby. Nikki was one of those Goku girls who decorated her binder with drawings of big-eyed anime boys, shirtless, chubby and often embracing, and this was like bringing her pictures to life. Sudden heat had filled the air as if the tree had flashed into flame. Brandon had never thought he was bi, and yet he'd found he liked this play, stuffing food into Zack's eager mouth while Nikki encouraged them.

Zach had been maybe a nanosecond away from creaming his jeans, but then the warning bell had rung. Still, they had lingered, panting like puppies, all of them hot as newborn stars.

Sitting here now in Health and Science, gazing out at the greenery, Brandon wondered what might have happened had they gone on with their play. He'd been dreaming about a "Nikki" all summer, but a "Zach" had never crossed his mind. And, "erotic eating" -- for lack of a better descriptive term -- had definitely never been on the menu. They had finally agreed to obey the bell, but Brandon wasn't sure they were saved.

"...An example of contagious obesity is that children raised by obese parents are likely to be obese themselves."

Carlos muttered, "An' children raised by stupid parents are likely to be Mr. Mortimers, which 'proves' stupidity is contagious."

Brandon glanced at Travis: he seemed to be taking notes, but was working on another story, part of a Beastworld episode that he and Brandon were going to vid. Tommy, of course, would be in it, and so would Ro and Kelvin, along with Danny and Carlos; a band of mutant terrorists who battled the evil Beastmaster and his plan for a planet of worker slaves.

It had been an interesting week, even without what had happened at lunch. Or what had almost happened... whatever that might have been.

Public school was fascinating, as Mr. Spock would have said; like a mission to a strange new world. Maybe the school itself was a joke in terms of actual education, but the people in it could fill several books, and writing class was priceless.

Brandon had read *The Encourager Clowns*, his satire story assignment, and total silence had followed. Mr. Akida had sat at his desk with no apparent reaction, though some of the students were watching him and waiting for a cue. Travis had only smiled, the way he'd looked that day on the bus when Brandon hadn't known where to sit. Brandon had wondered what was wrong, and sweat had suddenly sheened his face. Standing there at the front of the room, he'd felt as if he was totally naked... naked and maybe obese. Then, Mr. Akida had spoken:

"That, Mr. Williams, is the kind of applause that most of us who call ourselves writers will only dream of getting. You have left your audience stunned. Perhaps even shocked and dismayed. But, more than that, you have made them *think*... which is no small accomplishment in a culture where thinking is not encouraged. Whether they will admit it or not, you have planted a seed of doubt in their minds, which may grow into healthy skepticism and cause them to question so-called 'facts' instead of ignorantly accepting and perpetuating them. And, you have offended a few. That is also important, for how can a story be socially-conscious *unless* it offends someone?"

Then he had laughed. "It also takes a lot of courage to spit in the face, so to speak, of a clown when everyone else is enjoying the show. Including the refreshments. Writers have been imprisoned for less. Some have even been executed. Congratulations, Mr. Williams, you have earned an A."

Travis had started clapping, followed by Bosco and Rex. Finally the rest of the class had joined in. It had lasted so long that Security buzzed to ask if help was needed. Then Travis had read his story, standing up as big as a beast and too mookin' phat to be denied. Of course his piece was about being fat, a "day in the life" sort of thing; a day that was filled with ignorant hate, mostly from people who thought they were "good." He could have written an angry story; he might have tried for sympathy; but instead he chose to tell a tale about an average and likable boy of no particular color or race whose day was worse than The Elephant Man's... not because he was fat but because other people hated him for it.

It should have gotten the same reaction of stunned and brain-frozen silence, but the kids weren't going to be caught again and gave him a standing ovation. Security was becoming annoyed.

Mr. Akida had let it go on and waited a moment to speak:

"We are blessed with some truly great writers this year. They give me hope for the future. And the future of any society is always in the hands of its youth. As Mr. White has demonstrated, a story does not have to slap your face to make a satirical statement. While Mr. Williams went for your throats, Mr. White appealed to your hearts. Mr. Williams left you angry, feeling, perhaps, that you were fools to be taken in by 'colonels and clowns,' duped into fighting their fast-food wars and paying for the privilege. Mr. White, on the other hand, has hopefully left you saddened by pointing out an 'acceptable' wrong; an injustice condoned by society and encouraged by misinformation, self-serving junk-science and hate propaganda... exactly the same sort of propaganda that has in the past bred the burning of 'witches,' holy wars, and genocide. Congratulations, Mr. White, our second A this morning."

Also not surprisingly, Rex had written about being little, smaller than average for his age, the opposite of Travis's tale. His story was mostly anecdotes, like the pelican signs at the Boardwalk: *You have to be as tall as me to ride the roller-coaster.*

The class had relaxed and enjoyed this story -- of safety belts that couldn't be tightened, of child-seats at restaurants, and waiters bringing junior menus -- and laughter had lightened the atmosphere. Rex's style was a little rough, but he still received a lot of applause, and though he only got a B it seemed to be more than he'd expected.

And, maybe it wasn't surprising that Bosco had written of kids in the past, of how they'd invented a lot of cool things... the Frisbee, (tossing pie plates), Hula Hoops (from barrel bands), skateboards (made from roller skates), and the original Sting Ray bike (built from salvaged junk). The same applied to clothing styles.

But all these inventions were stolen from kids and "invented" by adults. To be sold (of course) to other kids who assumed adults invented them. This might have been a fact of life, an acceptable sort of thievery where adults were taking the credit (and profit) for things invented by kids. There wasn't much you could do about it -- kids had always been exploited -- but now these things, the toys, the clothes, the practical means of transportation, had to be made in factories and sold for money in stores.

Or they just weren't cool.

The irony in Bosco's tale was a boy in the cutoffs he'd styled himself, riding the skate he'd invented himself, and getting dissed by other kids who were wearing "Beachcombers" they'd bought in stores and cruising factory boards.

Mr. Akida had made a few comments, clueing the class about exploitation; how kids made billions for industries by buying the clothes they were told to buy, as well as the toys, the games and food... and now the body image.

Bosco had gotten an A.

A girl had raised her hand to say there was nothing kids could do about it: they couldn't vote, they had no power, and no one ever listened to them.

Mr. Akida responded by telling a tale about bubble gum: back in the 1970s, a kid had started a rumor that a certain brand contained spider's eggs. In weeks that rumor was nationwide -- long before the internet -- and the company was in trouble. It had to start an ad campaign convincing kids this wasn't true, which cost it millions of dollars.

Mr. Akida had added, "No one listens to kids you say? A million-dollar industry was virtually brought to its knees by kids! *Billions* of dollars are spent every year to make you want to buy new things. ...And whether you need them or not. You are being taught to buy and consume from the moment you watch your first TV show."

He'd paused to smile at Bosco. "To make your own things is not to consume, instead it is to conserve and recycle."

Then he had turned to the girl. "You say you have no power, young woman? Every one of you in this room has the mightiest power on earth today... the power of money and how you spend it. Read the labels on your clothing. Not the brand... which is often the only reason you bought it... but where those articles were made. The labels you seldom read. Often your clothes, your shoes and toys, your computer parts and video games, are made by children younger than you who can never afford to buy what they make. A child who works in a sweat-shop cannot go to school and better himself. He may survive on his few cents a day, but his life is dependent on you. In effect, you have made him your slave. That is obviously wrong, and perhaps some day you will right that wrong. You have that choice because you have power."

"How?" another girl had asked.

"That may seem like a complex question, but most such questions seem complex because they are *meant* to seem that way by people who don't want you to ask them. The busses in Montgomery, Alabama were not desegregated because someone solved a complex question of Civil Rights and morality; a question of if it was right or wrong that a black woman had to give up her seat if a white man wanted to sit. Those busses were desegregated because of a boycott by average people that cost the company thousands of dollars. *That* is the power you have, young people, the power to say that something is wrong and you won't accept, support, or buy it."

Mr. Akida had smiled again. "We have heard four excellent stories today which comment upon our society. We have been taught to listen to clowns. We have also been taught to hate people simply because of their size or weight. And, we are taught we must buy what we want, and consume more things than we actually need."

"But, some things are cool," a boy had protested.

"Some things *are* cool," agreed Mr. Akida. "I came to this country myself to have things, as well as the time to enjoy them. But, always ask yourself *why* you want something... a pair of shoes, a video game, or a body-image. And *why* do you think that something is cool? Are the jeans you are wearing comfortable? Or did you only buy them because of the name on a strip of cloth or a bit of leather? Now they will make more jeans like that... perhaps uncomfortable jeans... simply because you have chosen to buy them."

Mr. Akida had laughed. "You have probably paid eighty dollars for *five* dollars worth of blue denim canvas and a label or tag which cost a penny."

Rex had spoken up. "Isn't there a law against that? Like, making too much profit?"

"To a very limited extent, and seldom actually enforced. But, it is not completely profit. There is the cost of manufacture... even if only slave wages to a third-world child in a sweat-shop. The major expense is advertising: it costs a company millions of dollars to make you want to buy those jeans."

A chubby boy had laughed. "An' they gotta pay those skinny models."

Mr. Akida had nodded. "That is also expensive; magazines and television, and the internet. There are similar jeans at discount stores, and because they are not widely advertised they cost only twenty dollars."

"I got a pair of those," said a boy, blushing when snickers had rippled the room.

"That took courage," said Mr. Akida.

Rex had laughed. "It takes a lot more to wear 'em to school!"

"Because they're not cool," said a girl.

Mr. Akida had nodded again. "Now apply these ideas to how you look... your bodies, not your clothes. Who decides what a cool look is? Who *teaches* you what a cool look is... and also teaches you what is not? Your peers, you think? But who teaches them? Look at Brandon and Bosco. Both are blond and have blue eyes and resemble each other in many ways except for a difference in weight. If these young men were strangers to you... perhaps you saw them at a beach... who would you say looks cooler?"

The class had gone silent a moment or two, no one wanting to look uncool by actually speaking their mind, but then a girl had raised her hand.

"We've been taught that Brandon looks cooler because..." she blushed. "Bosco is fat." Then she giggled. "But I think Bosco is cuter."

"I do, too," said Mr. Akida. "But I'm from a place where kids are skinny because they don't have enough to eat, not because they think it looks cool or were taught it was healthy."

Now, Brandon gazed out at the sunlit trees while Mr. Mortimer droned on and on about the uncoolness of being fat. But his wearisome words and sterile statistics didn't seem to offend anyone, or even make them think.

Brandon's mind wandered among the trees as they drooped in the mid-September heat. There was no shortage of story ideas -- socially-conscious or otherwise -- to be found in public school. The week had been like a string of vignettes, and Wednesday had been interesting.

It had been in the cafeteria: Rex was sitting next to Brandon, stuffing himself with mashed potatoes, bean burritos, tamale pie, and washing it down with a chocolate shake. He was following Tommy's gainer advice, and had gained two pounds since Brandon's party. (His mother had let him sleep over, and he'd spent Sunday morning in Brandon's room, accepting a muzzy hangover as part of the process of getting "growed up," having breakfast with Brandon and Tommy -- sausage, eggs, and hash-browns -- and watching Cartoon Network.)

"I think Jason's in trouble," Rex had said.

Brandon looked up from his fish sticks, which were soggily breaded, greasily fried, and probably packed enough mercury to fill a dozen thermometers. But a rumor said there was beer in the batter and fish sticks were now in deadly demand. Brandon suspected the story was beans, but there had been fights over fish sticks when supplies had run low, and a boy had even been stabbed. The dean had denied the rumor, of course, denouncing it over the P.A. system and pleading for "peace and tolerance," but nothing was really believed in this school until the dean denied it.

Jason never ate with the beasts, usually taking a corner table over by the garbage cans, a place reserved for geeks and nerds... not to mention flies. Five big dudes surrounded him now; a couple of jocks from the football team and a trio of skinheads, including Joe Slater... who still believed in the Aryan race despite the fact it didn't exist. He'd tried to "save" Brandon and Bosco last week, reminding them -- duh! -- they were blue-eyed and blond. (His eyes were brown.) He'd also said they'd been chosen by God to exterminate the "mud-people races" and other threats to "real men," including Jews and gays. Bosco had said he was full of beans, while Brandon had called him a mooked-up mook, which had ended the salvation session. Joe had muttered, "Traitors will be dealt with."

Now he seemed to be dealing with Jason, as if being fat was inferior, too... or maybe a threat to "real men." It had probably been a spontaneous thing -- the dudes just going to dump their leftovers -- but now they were making Jason eat them.

"That sucks!" Zach had said.

Nikki had frowned. "Aren't you guys going help him?"

"Why should we?" said Carlos. "He never wants to hang with us."

"Him an' his dumb-ass diet," said Danny.

"He ain't lost no weight I can see," observed Kelvin.

Travis had sighed. "Guess we should give him some backup."

"Where's the security guard?" asked Rex.

"He won't do anything," said Danny. "They're only bullying a fat kid."

"Well," said Bosco. "Normally I'm a lover, but..."

191

Other kids were watching, most with smirks and snickers, but silence had settled over the room as the beasts got up and went to Jason, who sat with chocolate cake on his face.

"Oooo," said one of the jocks, a senior. "Here come the bad blubber-boys!"

"I could resent that," said Kelvin. "But, I don't."

Joe Slater scowled. "You people bring race into everything!"

"Excuse me?" said Travis. "I just brought myself." He glanced at some books that one of the seniors had set on the table. "You doing anything important?"

"Huh?" said the dude. "...No..."

"Then you'll wanna get these." Travis tossed the books in a garbage can.

"You fat...!"

"Save the drama for your mamma," said Travis, looking as big as a tank. Then he smiled at Joe. "See? It's not about race."

"*Buenos dias*, dickwads," said Carlos.

"This is none of you guyses business!" cried Joe.

Carlos smiled. "Then maybe you wanna keep it that way."

"This ain't about race!"

"Yeah it is," said Brandon. "The human race... real men."

"And real women," added Nikki.

"Yeah," said Danny Little-Wing. "And you're not human anymore 'cause you chose to de-evolve."

Brandon had nodded. "*You've* become the mud people by dragging yourselves back into it."

Rex had looked ready to snatch Joe's books and add them to the garbage can... which, Brandon noticed, included "the book." Joe grabbed them fast. "Traitors will be dealt with!"

Brandon had smiled. "Then I'd worry if I were you. You're a traitor to all good human beings."

Finally, one of the seniors had laughed... the one who still had ungarbaged books. "We were just punkin' him, dudes. We didn't mean nothin'."

"It might have meant something to him," said Danny.

Travis had added, "'Little boys throw stones at frogs in sport, but

192

the frogs die in earnest.' ...That's Plutarch, a real man."

A moment of silence had followed. The jocks were big and beefy, but Travis and Danny massed a lot more. Kelvin looked like a muscular Panther sizing up a white-tiger gang, and Bosco looked somehow dangerous because he only looked amused. Brandon had never been much of a fighter, but found himself measuring Joe. But then the seniors walked away, leaving Joe and his posse alone.

Travis said, "Go peddle your hate to some other fools who don't have the brains to think for themselves."

Joe and his followers left.

Jason glared up from the wreckage of plates and half-eaten food on his table. "I didn't ask you guys for nothing!"

"You're welcome," said Danny, then added, "Next time you'll get an abundance of nothing."

Now, sitting here in Health and Science, Brandon studied Jason: he seemed to be the only kid who hated being fat.

"...Every year," the teacher droned on, "there are 300,000 deaths in America because of obesity."

Travis murmured to Brandon, "I've had enough of this stupid shit." He raised his hand.

Mr. Mortimer looked surprised; no one asked questions in Health and Science. "...Yes?"

"Those statistics were never objectively proven. The original study they're based on never mentioned other health-risks fat people might have, like drinking, smoking, or drug use. ...Including diet drugs. Especially all those sold on TV that never have to be tested. That study also never mentioned excessive dieting, yo-yo dieting, or diet itself as contributing factors to death or poor health. Or depression or stress... like from getting dissed all the time. None of those things were studied, and their effects on average size people were never compared to fat ones."

Mr. Mortimer blinked like a deer caught in headlights. Then he cleared his throat. "These are facts in your *Health and Science book*," he said in an almost astonished voice, as if Travis had spit on a Bible.

Travis raised an eyebrow. "So why isn't one of those 'facts' that life expectancy in the U.S. is now the highest it's ever been? Isn't life expectancy one of the most accurate measures of health in any society?"

"...Well, yes," said Mr. Mortimer. "But life expectancy statistics are also based on infant and childhood mortality rates, which are very low in America. Babies are born healthy and therefore don't... er... pass away."

"Agreed," said Travis. "But those statistics are also based on how long people live; and the Baby Boom generation, who grew up eating all the 'wrong food,' and many of whom are 'obese,' are living longer and healthier than any generation before."

"It's been projected that may change," said Mr. Mortimer. He seemed to study Travis's bulk spilling out of the desk. "Because of childhood obesity."

"Because more kids are fat?" asked Travis. "Or, because of how they got fat?"

The teacher blinked again. "I don't understand."

"I'll try to keep it simple," said Travis. "Isn't it true that *unbiased* studies have shown that fat people who don't eat a lot of junk-food, get moderate exercise and are basically happy... meaning not depressed or always stressed from constantly being hated-on... are just as healthy and live just as long as skinny or average size people? Isn't it also true that other unbiased studies have shown that average size people who eat lots of junk-food, don't exercise, and are stressed or depressed, often die sooner than other people?"

"I... haven't heard of such studies."

Travis smiled. "Maybe because they're not in your book. and some teachers just teach what they've been taught... which is junk educa-tion. ...Would you say it's possible that all this concern about obesity is only an example of medicalizing a lifestyle, behavior and physical appearance that's now being taught is incorrect? A lifestyle, behavior and physical look that goes against the System's values... values the System wants us to live by... which often infringe on, restrict or deny the rights of individuals to life, liberty, and the pursuit of happiness?"

"...That's an... interesting... supposition, Mr.... er, White. But..." Mr. Mortimer stared around. For the first time his class was listening

194

to him and it seemed to be scary.

Travis went on, "Would you also say it's possible that 'health' and diet industries are actually doing most of the research supposedly proving fat is bad, because it's very profitable to make people want to lose weight or stay skinny?"

"...Well, again that's an interesting..."

"Didn't President Eisenhower warn the American people in 1961 that the U.S. might be eventually ruled by a military-industrial complex where science and research were controlled and funded by self-serving private corporations whose only motive was profit?"

"...President Eisenhower?" said Mr. Mortimer.

"The President before Kennedy."

"I know!" said Mr. Mortimer, flushing a little. "But, this is Health and Science class."

"Nah," said Travis. "It's health-nazi hype and *junk* science class encouraging mindless conformity and xenophobic hate."

Snickers and laughter broke out in the room, and Mr. Mortimer flushed again. "Mr. ...er, White. The information in this book has been compiled by the government to shape your way of thinking for life."

"I know," said Travis. "Which scares me a lot more than being fat."

TWENTY-ONE

"C'mon," said Tommy. "I'll buy dessert at Baskin-Robbins."

"Get your allowance back?" asked Brandon.

"Nah, but Da Beast know how to survive."

It was late afternoon, around five o'clock, and they'd just left the Mission Street McDonalds toting their skateboards under their arms. Brandon paused to pat his tummy, which bulged out over his low-riding jeans and bobbed a bit as he walked. "You bought me two Quarter-Pounders with cheese, plus a super-size Coke and fries. You must be mowing a lot of lawns."

"Nah, I been making fat vids."

"How does that make money?"

"They're private shows," said Tommy. "I post previews for free, but you gotta pay to see the whole thing. Plus I do special requests. Pays hella better than mowing lawns."

"But, what if weirdos are watching? Pedophiles or predators?"

"Their money's as good as anyone else's. But most of my fans are kids."

"It still seems kinda perverted."

Tommy shrugged. "Perverted people pervert everything. And now they're perverting being fat, which is one of the most normal things in the world. ...Um, you're not freaked?"

"Nah," said Brandon. "I got an IM the other night from some old guy who saw my pic and wanted me for a gay teen site... 'as long as I didn't get too chubby.'"

"Gays are some of the worst fat-haters; like, 'hate on me 'cause I'm gay and that's wrong, but I can hate you 'cause you're fat.'"

196

Brandon looked down at his tumescent tummy. "You sure you're not encouraging me?"

Tommy laughed. "Maybe a little. But you look happy when you're eating, which makes me happy, too." He burped, and added, "You know I gotta get fatter, but *you* didn't have to eat all that."

Brandon smiled. "Always happy to make you happy, but I hope you win your fat war soon or I'm gonna need all new jeans."

They carried their boards across the street, and Tommy laughed again. "What you said about Nikki and Zach and what you did at lunch today? Maybe you wanna be encouraged?"

"I don't wanna try to steal Zach's girl, if that's what you're talking about. I like the dude."

"A lot if you fed him an' rubbed his belly."

"It wasn't like that! ...For me, I mean."

"You didn't get sprung?"

"...Because Nikki was making us do it."

"She zap you with an erection ray?"

"I told you, man, it was like we were anime characters acting out her drawings."

Tommy grinned. "More like her fantasies. But you like Nikki, huh?"

"I can't help it," sighed Brandon. "And when I see her feeding Zach... Oh, never mind."

"Dis Da Beast you're talking to, Bucky. Me understand those feelings."

Brandon sighed again. "So, what am I supposed to do? Stop hang-ing with Zach and Nikki? Like that old song, *Jessie's Girl?*"

"Why? I thought you liked them. And doing what you did today underneath that tree."

"That part scares me a little."

"It takes a brave man to admit when he's scared."

"Did you ever feed Zach?"

"Tons of times at the Boardwalk. He'd send me out for burgers, then we'd go behind the softee machine and I'd stuff him till he was ready to pop."

"Does that have a Freudian meaning?"

197

"There are exploding cigars."

"You think everyone should be fat?"

"Troy thinks everyone should have muscles... as long as they don't have more than him.""

"Um, did you ever hug Zach?"

"Like you hugged me?"

"Just asking for information. Information. Information."

Tommy smiled. "I think you mean something more than a hug. Like, deeper and more meaningful. Could we call it a cuddle?"

"...Guess we could," said Brandon. "At least between you and me."

"Wouldn't that be you and I?"

"Technically, but it's archaic."

"Look at it this way," said Tommy. "Would you wanna be thirty and wonder about what you might have missed? ...Like all the things you could have done when it was the time to do 'em."

"Did you ever want to cuddle somebody?"

"I assume you mean of the same sex or the answer would be obvious."

"You may also assume that's a duh."

"I could cuddle with Bosco."

"...I think I could, too. ...But, why?"

Tommy thought for a moment. "There's something different about him and it's something you wanna get close to... like, be a part of as much you can before that time gets away."

"I feel that way, too. ...Would you ever ask him?"

"I don't think I would."

"Why not?"

"Because he's innocent."

"But, I'm sure he's had sex," said Brandon. "With a girl, I assume. And probably more than one. So how can he be innocent?"

Tommy shrugged. "I'd feel like Mrs. Robinson."

"You mean you'd be seducing him?"

"I mean I'd feel like I was. ...Like, even if he wanted to, it woulda been my idea."

"I don't understand," said Brandon.

Tommy considered. "I don't think he thinks about stuff like that... Bosco, I mean... like anybody would want him that way. ...Bet he don't have a mirror in his room."

"Is that significant?" asked Brandon.

"In this culture yes. Because we've been taught we need mirrors to maintain an acceptable image to an image-obsessive society. But it would be natural if Bosco didn't."

"Why?"

"'Cause he's never been taught he needed one. ...Also applies to innocence; he's never been taught he's not."

"Is that why you never asked me to cuddle? 'Cause you think I'm innocent?"

"Sorta."

"But what about jacking-off?"

That's just jacking-off. ...And you're older than me; if you wanted to cuddle *you* should have asked."

"I would have felt like Mrs. Robinson."

"Did you ever think about asking?"

"Not till I met Bosco. ...Which makes me kinda confused."

"Think about it over dessert. Just don't listen to all the voices."

"Which one should I listen to?"

"The little guy with the halo sitting on your shoulder."

Brandon paused on the sidewalk. "Speaking of dessert, I just thought of something."

"All the time you wasted not asking me to cuddle?"

"Oh, shut up." Brandon pointed up the street. "There's your school."

"Yeah, so?"

"Did you ever notice that all around are nothing but junk-food joints? Like, there's a McDonalds, a Burger King, a Taco Bell and a Jack In The Box. And there's a Wendys, a Baskin-Robbins, a Pizza Hut, and an AM-PM. And they're all around your school."

"Saves a lot of walking."

"But they can't put up a cigarette ad, or a beer or liquor billboard for at least three blocks around a school... like that matters. But they can surround it with junk-food joints. And none of that stuff is sup-posedly healthy."

Tommy shrugged. "About fifty people get killed every day in car accidents. But they don't stop selling cars, do they? Or telling people how cool they are and making them want to buy one. And cars pollute the environment so they're unhealthy for everybody."

"Beast has a point."

Tommy pointed to another billboard. "Maybe that's supposed to protect us."

Brandon glanced at the towering sign:

CHILDHOOD OBESITY, DON'T TAKE IT LIGHTLY!

He'd seen the same ad on TV many times, but like most public service commercials he'd never paid any attention. "Does that bother you?"

"Did those anti-pot ads bother you? Like, 'Don't Let Your Childhood Go Up In Smoke?'"

"Which I almost did," said Brandon. "But I thought they were lame. Most of those public-service things are. They try to make something seem uncool, but they do it in such a stupid way it only makes kids want do it."

"Yeah," agreed Tommy. "And the more they try to make fat uncool, the more some kids will wanna be fat. There's more gainer kids on the web every day."

"Kinda like Prohibition."

"Huh?"

"Like, back in the 1920s when they made alcohol illegal. It only made drinking cool."

"Oh yeah," said Tommy. "And all those gangsters got hella rich."

"Just like the colonels and clowns today."

"Don't forget the diet mob."

"Like supplying both sides in a war," said Brandon. "They get people's money one way or the other."

"Sometimes both ways," said Tommy. "Just like you said, eat all the time but don't get fat." He glanced at the billboard again. "Right now all those do is say it's okay to dis and hate fat kids."

200

They entered the ice cream shop. "I'll have a small sundae," said Brandon. "Blueberry. And a small lemonade, since I don't have a fat war to win."

Tommy ordered a large hot fudge with a big lemonade for himself, and they took the stuff to a table. There were several kids at another table, fifth or sixth-graders, Brandon guessed. Two of them were super-size with bellies spilling over their jeans, but they didn't seem shy about it. The fattest kid wore a tight tank-top with his boy-breasts lolling out on each side. His tan suggested he often wore less, so he obviously wasn't a hider.

Tommy noticed where Brandon was looking. "Most fat kids are normal... or would be if haters would let 'em."

"I know you're normal, but what do you mean?"

"Like, being fat is part of us, and most of us don't think much about it."

"Until somebody tells you it's bad."

"Or makes it erotic because it's forbidden. Which is why I'm making money."

"I was thinking about the other dudes with them."

"The average size kids?" said Tommy. "Like, they don't care if their friends are fat."

"Yeah."

Tommy spooned ice cream. "Some kids still manage to think for themselves. They don't need TV, teachers or billboards to tell them who or what they should like. Or to chose their friends by the pound. ...They gave us a test in back in kindergarten. They showed us two drawings, one of a fat kid and another one of an average kid. They asked which one we'd wanna play with."

Brandon sipped lemonade. "What happened?"

"Everybody but me picked the average size kid. Even the other fat kids."

"Zot?"

"The drawing of the average kid made him look like Mr. Cool with designer jeans and a big friendly smile. But the drawing of the fat kid made him look like a geek in a striped T-shirt and Mickey Mouse shorts. All he needed was one of those beanies with a propeller on top. And he looked about ready to cry any second. Like, if you just *thought* the word fat, he'd bust into tears and spaz-out." Tommy laughed. "Even I didn't wanna play with him."

"So, why did you choose him?" asked Brandon.

"I felt sorry for him. Like, maybe if I could cheer him up and get him into some normal clothes, he might have been cool after all."

"Yeah," said Brandon. "I read about where they did that with dolls. They showed a bunch of mostly white kids a white doll and a black one. Then they asked the kids which doll was more handsome. All the kids picked the white doll. Even the black kids. Then they showed them a movie with cool black kids. Then all the kids picked the black doll."

Tommy gulped lemonade. "That's subliminal programming. Influencing people with images to make them think how you want them to think. Ever notice in ads for losing weight, the 'before' picture always looks unhappy?"

"Hey, that's right. Like, a smile makes a lot of difference."

Tommy smiled like a happy cherub. "Starting to get the pic?"

"You are who they say you are... 'they' being those in control, and the ones making money." He glanced at the other kids. "Like, make that fat dude... or you... the star of some cool movie, and fat kids would be cool overnight."

"Even if some of them weren't."

Brandon glanced up as a boy came in. "Speaking of looking unhappy, *he* keeps saying he's on a diet, so what's he doing in here?"

Tommy looked around. "Oh, *him*. Now, he's not a normal fat kid."

"You know him?" asked Brandon.

Tommy spooned more ice cream. "No more than I wanna. But I know what his problem is. ...Why? You know him?"

"No more than I wanna," said Brandon. "That's Jason from my P.E. class. Got him in World History and Health and Science, too."

"Oh, *that's* the mook you told me about. Figures. He comes here all the time."

"Funny," said Brandon, sipping his drink. "He's always hating on himself. He's shy as mook about his body, like he should be a hider,

202

but he always wears clothes that *don't* hide his fat and actually make him look fatter. ...'Course, maybe that's the biggest size he could find in an Area 51 shirt."

"Nah," said Tommy. "That's an outward sign of his problem. For normal fat kids it's normal if your fat peeks out of your shirt, but he lets his fat show 'cause he hates being fat."

"Zot?"

"It's like wearing a sign that says Please Don't Hate Me."

"But that wouldn't do any good," said Brandon. "It would be like an invitation to haters... like waving a flag in front of a bull, to use a clichéd expression."

"Ya think?" said Tommy.

"Bucky to Beast, I'm confused again. Jason says he's obese and he's trying to lose weight, so why would he want to get hated more?"

Tommy glanced at Jason, who had ordered a small strawberry sundae. "Want Da Beast to illustrate?"

"Illustrate what?"

"Jason's problem... and it's gonna look cruel. You gotta go along with me. No matter what happens don't stop me. Okay?"

"...Okay."

Jason started for a table, his sundae and Coke on a tray. Tommy turned around again. "Hey, obese pig!"

Brandon stiffened in surprise. Jason's cheeks turned pink, but he ignored Tommy.

"...Oh. Hi, Brandon."

"Hey, Jason," said Brandon, not knowing what else to say.

Tommy looked disgusted. "Hey, obese pig! Your fat obese belly is hanging out."

Jason looked nervous and tugged at his shirt.

"Give it up, fatso!" sneered Tommy. "You're *way* too obese to hide all your fat! Even fat kids think you're obese!"

Brandon almost told Tommy to shut the mook up, but Tommy gave him a glance before adding, "Get your fat ass over here and stick your fat face in the pig trough, fatty!"

"Go to hell," said Jason, though without much anger. "This is frozen yogurt and Diet Coke. I'm trying to lose weight."

Tommy laughed. "You never will, you obese tub of fat! 'Cause you're a fat obese pig and can't stop stuffing your fat obese face! Get your fat ass over here or I'll start yelling obese real loud!"

Again, Brandon almost protested, but Tommy kicked him under the table as Jason came over hesitantly.

"Give him lots of room, Brandon," said Tommy. "He's so obese he can hardly get behind the table!" Then he added as Jason sat down, "I know you want a *lot* more than that! You wanna stuff your big fat belly till you're so obese you can't even walk!"

"No I don't," Jason said weakly.

"Eat, fat pig!" ordered Tommy. "Stuff it down or I'll start yelling obese blubber tub and everybody will stare at you! ...Hey, obese pig, how much money you got?"

"I don't have any more."

"Don't lie to me, lardo, give it here!"

"...No."

"Shut up and stuff your fat obese face! ...And I said give it here, or I'll tear off your shirt and you'll have to go out on the street with all your obesity showing!"

"Tom..." Brandon began, but was kicked again.

Jason, his mouth full of sundae, pulled twenty dollars out of a pocket. Tommy shoved the bill at Brandon. "Buy him a *big* banana split. With everything on it and extra whipped cream!"

Jason looked ready to cry. "No! I'll get even more obese."

"Shut up, fat pig!" ordered Tommy. "I'm gonna *make* you get more obese so everybody will hate you more!"

Brandon stood up, not touching the money. "Tommy..."

"Look at him, man, he wants it so much 'cause he's nothing but a fat obese pig!" Tommy faced Jason again. "Eat, blubber-boy! 'Cause if you don't stuff your big obese belly I'm gonna start yelling obese!"

"I gotta go to the bathroom!" Jason got up and practically ran.

"Shit, Tommy!" snapped Brandon. "The mook is wrong with you, man? That totally sucks! Let's get out of here!" He threw down his spoon. "I just lost my appetite!"

Tommy shrugged. "But he's gonna be so disappointed if I don't make him eat a lot more. And I got him sprung, which is why he ran

204

to the bathroom."

"...The mook are you talking about?"

Tommy spooned up the last of his sundae. "That's what he *wants*. And he'll hang around here till someone else does it to him on the real. There's plenty of haters."

"That's..."

"Perverted?" Tommy suggested.

Brandon sat down and slid the bill under Jason's Coke. "...Just like at lunch the other day. Remember I told you what happened? When those big dudes tried to make him eat? And he acted pissed-off 'cause we stopped them."

"Does Bucky begin to see a light?"

"...As long as somebody makes him eat, it's not his fault he's fat?"

"He prefers 'obese,'" said Tommy. "For reasons already covered."

"Are there a lot of fat kids like him?"

"There's gonna be a lot more with all this anti-obesity shit. Some want to be called hater names."

"Jason *likes* getting hated?"

"Nah, I'm sure he hates it. But his problem is he hates himself more, so he thinks he deserves to be hated."

"Zot?"

"Nobody likes him because he's 'obese.' I'm sure his mom tells him that every day."

"Double zot," said Brandon.

"He doesn't have any friends, but at least he thinks he knows why."

"But he might be cool in his own way. Like that Area 51 shirt... he might know a lot about aliens. That would still make him a geek to some people. ...Like, I'm a geek to some people."

"So am I," said Tommy. "Hard as that might be to believe. Everybody's a geek to somebody. But we know some people aren't gonna like us no matter who we are."

"'Cause we have self-esteem?"

"Bucky wins a big fat cigar. ...But Jason doesn't have self-esteem. Somebody beat it out of him. If I had to guess I'd say his mom, starting at an early age. Then the haters finished the job. He's used to being hated... or just not liked... because he's 'obese.' But, what if he got skinny and people *still* didn't like him? There's a dude on the web like that: he was fat all his life till he turned sixteen an' got part of his stomach cut out. He lost all his fat but he still can't make friends. His 'problem' wasn't being fat, his problem is he's boring! He was boring when he was fat, and now he's twice as boring 'cause all he wants to talk about is how good he thinks he feels being skinny."

"Thinks he is?" said Brandon.

Tommy fondled his breasts. "Different strokes for different folks, but I wouldn't feel good being skinny."

"How would you know, you've never been skinny."

"I've never had a hemorrhoid either, but I'm pretty sure I wouldn't like one."

"That dude you described sounds like those kids they bring to school to talk about being former druggies or alcoholics."

"Like your uncle who comes for Christmas and bores everybody with the 'evils of drinking' and how good he feels since he stopped."

"Yeah," said Brandon. "Even dad says nobody's more boring than a former alcoholic."

"Unless it's a former fat person," said Tommy. "They'll probably start doing that... bring kids who lost weight to bore us at school about how 'cool' it is to be skinny."

"Couldn't you talk to Jason? Professionally, I mean?"

"I'm good, but I'm not that good. Jason's been hated for fourteen years, probably starting with his mom who's been telling him he'll never have friends as long as he's obese. And now he's gotten to the point where being abused for being obese is actually exciting, even though he hates it. We're talking major therapy now, and that would have to include his mom 'cause she's established a pattern, too... of dissing Jason because he's fat. Even assuming she thinks she loves him... that she's doing it for 'his own good'... she's mooked up her mind along with his. She's used to mentally battering him and he's used to being battered, and they both think he deserves it 'cause all the haters say he does."

"So, you can't help him?" said Brandon.

206

"Not with his mom in control... I am only twelve. I did try telling him once that if he'd stop listening to her... start fighting back like I do... he'd realize he *can* have friends; that people will like him for who he is; and some people aren't gonna like him no matter what he weighs." Tommy shrugged. "And if he doesn't start fighting back, he'll just keep hating himself."

"Till something snaps?" asked Brandon.

"He's wound too tight already," said Tommy. "Pardon the dead cliché."

TWENTY-TWO

"Woah!" puffed Travis, stopping Brandon's skateboard by dragging the toe of his sneak. He shook sweat drops from his dreads and mopped his face with the tail of his shirt, though he'd only been riding the board with Brandon's pushing providing the power.

The morning sun was growing hot, and Brandon was also starting to sweat. "Just asking for information," he puffed, "information, information," while tugging Travis' slipping jeans halfway up his enormous bottom, a chore he was growing accustomed to. "Do you know how much you weigh?"

"Dad put me on a truck scale just before we moved down here and I weighed 487," said Travis. "But I'm sure I'm at least 500 now; which, if you'll excuse the pun, is a nice round number." He patted his gigantic belly, making it wobble in waves. "Most of those kids who wanna gain weight fantasize about getting this fat, but they don't have a clue what it's really like, and they might not think it's so boss if they were." He wiped his face again. "It's not so much from eating a lot, it's mostly not getting enough exercise. I can't do push-ups 'cause I can't get my belly off the floor." He laughed. "And if I tried doing jumping-jacks I'd go *through* the floor."

"Could you lift weights?" asked Brandon.

"Don't see why not. I lift tons every day just getting around."

"I could ask Chad about using his bench. And you can swim in our pool. I read that's good exercise for..."

"People so fat they can barely walk?"

"...Well, yeah."

"Guess I could give it a try." Travis laughed again. "'Least I'd be a

208

fat boy with muscles."

"You must have hella muscles already from packing all your fat around."

Travis patted his blubber. "Guess they're under here somewhere."

"What about going for walks?"

"I usually do on the beach in the morning. Always take Ro along, too. But you get awful tired of being hated. Like in that story I wrote, sometimes you feel like the Elephant Man. And most of the people doing the hating would probably never say nigger... even if they wanted to. They think they're so mookin' enlightened, liberal and tolerant... *except* when it comes to fat kids. Then they're still lynching niggers. I know what it must have been like in the South before we got our Civil Rights."

Brandon nodded. "I never knew there were so many haters until I started paying attention."

"No reason you would," said Travis. "There's nothing to hate about you."

"Who hates the color beige?" said Brandon. "Nobody creams their jeans about it, but nobody hates it either." He helped Travis step off the board by providing a shoulder to lean on. Though he'd known Travis for nearly two weeks, he still often found himself surprised that Travis was no any taller than he and only his girth made him seem so huge. "Um, hypothetical question...?"

"Shoot."

"Say you weren't fat...?"

"Light-years ahead of you, Brandy. Some people would hate me because I'm black. Or not cool in some other way to their definition of cool."

"Or because you're smart."

"I'd blush but it wouldn't show." Travis looked around. "It's cool here. Like being out in the country. 'Cept I never been out in the country. Our church always sponsored a summer camp but they said I was too fat to go, and so was Roosevelt."

"Zot?"

"In good Christian words like, 'we wouldn't have fun.'"

"That sucks!" said Brandon. "Didn't they take handicapped kids?"

"In wheelchairs? Sure."

"Um, couldn't you and Ro...?"

"Go in wheelchairs? That wouldn't be fair to the handicapped kids. Like using a handicapped placard to get a parking space, and some real handicapped person might need it."

Brandon waved a hand around. "This is just Old Wharf Road, I wouldn't call it the country."

"Most things are relative."

Brandon looked down a tree-covered slope to a glimmering creek far below, its sunlit sparkle barely seen through interlocking branches and leaves. Bird-song filled this suburban forest, and squirrels chattered cheerfully. The air was sweet with the scents of late summer, resinous pine, fragrant wild flowers, and blackberry vines heavy with fruit. "Hard to believe we're only a mile from Capitola Mall."

"Yeah," agreed Travis. "It's like another planet to me. ...So, this is the place?"

Brandon pointed to a hand-carved sign nailed to a tree by a rusty mailbox. "That's what Bosco said: Tiki Island, Old Wharf Road."

Travis studied a narrow dirt lane that tunneled steeply downward beneath the overhanging trees. It was deeply rutted with tire tracks, and half washed-out by winter rains. "I'm way too fat to walk back up so I probably shouldn't go down."

"Bosco's got his van."

"But walking downhill is almost as hard. I can't see my feet, y'know. And I have to lean backward to balance my belly even more than I normally do." Travis shrugged. "I'm just too fat to go down there. Sorry to disappoint you."

"It's nothing you have to apologize for."

"I wouldn't to anyone else. But I wouldn't be here with anyone else."

"C'mon, Travis, give it a try."

Travis looked doubtful but said, "Aight. But I'm probably gonna lose my jeans."

"I'll pull 'em up if they fall off. Put your arm over my shoulders and let me carry the board."

"Take it slow and careful," said Travis. "If I start to fall, get out of the way."

"Never happen, man. We'll go down together or win the fight like the mutant boys of Beastworld. ...Ready?"

"Might as well lose my shirt."

"Here, let me help."

Like just about everything else, shedding his shirt was a struggle for Travis. Brandon helped him peel it off, then stripped off his own and tied them both around his waist. "Are you gonna be okay?"

Travis shrugged. "There's nothing wrong with me, I'm just too fat for this kinda stuff. It's like what you said about Bosco's board, I'm like trying to fly a tank."

"C'mon, it's time for us to fly."

The air grew cooler as they descended, smelling of pine and the creek far below, of mossy rocks and ferny places. The steep lane was in pretty sad shape, and muddy in spots from Thursday's rain. Travis slipped a couple of times but Brandon managed to steady him. As he had warned, Travis had to lean way back to counterbalance his belly as it plunged and rebounded and wobbled and quaked, and Brandon had to guide his feet by telling him where to step. Then they came to a big mud puddle extending across the road.

"Guess this is as far as I go," said Travis.

"Zot?" said Brandon. "This is nothing. I could jump... Oh."

Travis smiled. "Sure you could, but I can't."

"But..."

"It's nothing you have to feel sorry about. I'm just too fat for stuff like this. I'll wait here, aight? Munch some berries like a beast. You guys can pick me up in the van."

"But don't you wanna see Bosco's crib? You know it's gotta be bitchin' boss."

"'Course I do, but I can't. Face it, Brandon, I'm just too fat."

Brandon studied the chocolate-brown puddle. "It can't be very deep. And it's only a little mud. We can take off our shoes and roll up our jeans."

Travis shook his head. "It's only a little mud to *you*. To me it's an

211

ocean of quicksand. One step in there and I'd be stuck, and you'd need a crane to pull me out. I'll just wait here till you come back. It's pretty, man... all shady and cool. And more in the country then I've ever been." He laughed. "I can pretend I went to camp."

"But check it out," said Brandon. "There's some rocks along the bank. You can use 'em for stepping stones."

"But I can't see my feet."

"I'll walk beside you and tell you where to step. Keep your arm on my shoulder. ...Look, there's a branch you can grab."

"But it's not *important*, Brandon. And why should you get muddy for me?"

Brandon tossed his board across, then waded into the water, which came about to his ankles. "Too late now, I'm already muddy."

Travis shook his head again. "I think you're a little wack sometimes." Then he sighed. "Aight. Here goes. ...But, this is probably a mistake."

"Put your arm on my shoulder," said Brandon. "There, you're on the first rock. Now step with your other foot. ...A little more. ...Can you reach the branch?"

"Not yet... Shit! The rock's sinking! I'm gonna fall! Get out of the way!"

"No, man! Grab the branch!"

"Move goddammit! ...Let go of me!"

"No mookin' way! Grab the branch, Travis!"

"I got it," puffed Travis. "But it's breaking! Let go of me, fool, or you're gonna get hurt!"

"NO!" gasped Brandon, pouring sweat as he struggled to hold the enormous boy. "Get a grip, goddammit!"

Travis was panting but sounded calm as he tried to steady his bulk. "Aight. But it's gonna break. And the rock is gonna turn over. And you're hurting your back! Just let me fall. Like you said it's just mud."

"No," said Brandon. "Just one more step. ...Do it, dork!"

"And this branch is gonna *break!* ...You know how mookin' stupid this is?"

"I can't hold you up much longer! ...TRY, goddammit!"

"What's your problem, Brandon?"

"*You* right now! ...Reach out your mookin' foot, Travis! Give me a little help at least!"

"Brandon," puffed Travis. "You're gonna get hurt trying to help me. ...Yo, man, get on the real! I'm not some mutant Beastworld prince! I'm just a dude who's so freakin' fat I can't get across a little mud puddle! What's cool about that? ...You hear what I'm telling you? Now, get the hell out of my way!"

"TRY!" yelled Brandon. "Or I'll push your ass into that mud and we'll both never know if you could have made it!"

"Sure you just don't wanna get squished and you've been too shy to ask?"

"...What?"

"It's common fantasy for admirers, getting squished by a fat dude."

Brandon laughed. "I could barely breathe under Tommy; I'd look like Judge Doom in *Roger Rabbit* after the steamroller scene under you. And, considering the mud, I wouldn't find it arousing... assuming that's the implication."

"What about without the mud?"

"Let's file that for now and deal with the current situation."

Travis blew out a sigh. "Aight. Here goes..."

The next rock held, and so did the branch. Travis reached the other side and stood panting and dripping sweat while leaning on Brandon.

Brandon was also panting. "I guess... you gotta... kill me now."

"Why?" said Travis. "I gotta piss, and you can hold up my belly."

"Don't make me laugh, I don't have the breath."

"I wasn't making a funny."

"...Oh," said Brandon. "I, um, wondered about that."

"Wonder no more, wonder-boy." Travis glanced back at the puddle. "So, what the mook did that prove? You got me across a little mud puddle. ...But, thanks, I guess. ...You mooked up your shoes."

"I can wash 'em."

"How's your back?"

"I'll know tomorrow. Right now it's still working. ...You need to piss?"

"I can wait till we get to Bosco's."

"Don't ever wait!" snapped Brandon. "And, by the way, I *do* think you're cool despite your best efforts to prove me wrong."

"I don't have to be fat, y'know."

"People don't have to be haters either."

"That's a *non sequitur*. People don't have to be lots of things."

"But I always have to be Brandon."

"You won a great victory, Brandon. They'll write it down in history books: Brandon gets fat boy across mud puddle."

"You said that already. ...So, what do I do?"

"Just grab all the blubber you can, and lift. ...Heavy, ain't it?"

"Slippery too."

"Don't hurt your back. And get a good grip, this might take a while."

"You should have told me, Travis."

"I was hoping I'd just sweat it out."

"Don't ever do that again! Is there anything else I should know?"

"I'd move a little if I were you. I can't see it, therefore I can't aim it."

"Get serious, man," said Brandon. "What I'm saying is... well... like suppose you were epileptic? Or needed some kinda medicine? Or couldn't eat peanuts or something? You gotta tell me what you need. It's not fair if you don't."

"Fair to who? ...Or would that be whom?"

"To both of us. Friends are there for each other, but we gotta know our weaknesses."

"Very Beastworld. What's your weakness?"

"Maybe I ask too many questions."

"The answer is 42. ...Well, this is something you should know; how Travis takes a piss."

"Woah," said Brandon in spite of himself after hoisting Travis's belly. "Where is it?"

"In another dimension, except when we're in the pleasure dome."

"...Um... can you?"

"Sure, and frequently, but not in the way you know it, Jim." Travis laughed. "And since it's surrounded by fat... warm soft fat, if you wanna get literarily graphic... it's like getting massaged all the time, so it's kinda hard not to cream my jeans if I start having arousing thoughts."

"I've had a few accidents like that without being 'warmly and softly surrounded.'"

"Well, now you can pull up my jeans, again. Then you can tie my sneaks if they need it. ...And you can come over tonight and help me take a shower. Lift up my belly and wash underneath. Which, as you can probably guess, is also required after self-loving sessions and an occasional wet dream. ...Still wanna be friends?"

"Oh, shut up, man."

"Sure you're not an admirer?"

"Don't even go there!" snapped Brandon. "I'd like you if you looked like Kelvin, as long as you were still you."

"But I probably wouldn't be."

"Don't you think you deserve any friends?"

"Don't you think you deserve any normal friends?"

"Disregarding Tommy, you're the most normal person I've ever met." Brandon struggled with Travis's jeans. "It's not your fault you got this fat."

"Eeeeeh, wrong! It is my fault."

"Why?" asked Brandon. "'Cause you don't wanna take some pills all your life? Drugs that mook you up? Or have part of your stomach cut out? Or never be able to eat normally? ...And don't even talk about exercise! You think I'd wanna go for walks with haters dissing me all the time? People who call themselves normal and good, but who don't even have the... I don't know what... the brains, compasssion, or just decent feelings... to think there might be a reason you're fat. That it's even natural you're fat, besides being 'stupid and lazy.'"

"But what if I didn't have a reason? Lots of fat kids don't, y'know? They're just fat."

"So, why do they need a reason? Being fat isn't a crime."

"There's people who want to make it one, and they're working hard to do it."

"There's people who wanna put me in jail for riding my skate in front of their house. Or wearing sagger jeans. There's people who wanna drop bombs on kids. There's people who wanna exterminate Jews. Or Muslims, Christians, gays, or niggers."

Travis laughed. "You're getting good at saying that word; you don't hesitate anymore."

Brandon also laughed, straightening up and rubbing his back. "Tommy's been my friend all my life, and he's got a reason for being fat. There's all this food around all the time, and it takes off its clothes and jumps up and down and screams EAT ME NOW, BIG BOY!"

"Oh, shut up," chuckled Travis. "You're scaring the cute little squirrels."

"Take away their bushy tails and they're not cute, they're just rats in the trees. Take away all the hype about 'health' and you've just got assholes who have to hate, and preferably someone who can't fight back. Or people trying to make other people live the way they think they should. Not to mention companies making their bank accounts obese." Brandon tugged up Travis's jeans. "Do you think you're too fat?"

"What do you think?" asked Travis. "Based on what you've learned today."

"Are you happy being you?"

"I'm happy being me with you in the present place and time. ...Guess I have to kill you now."

Brandon laughed. "Then you'd lose a useful friend."

TWENTY-THREE

Both boys were out of breath again, Brandon from helping Travis walk by bearing a blubbery arm on his shoulders and one of his own around Travis – at least as much as possible -- by the time they'd descended the winding lane and reached the banks of Soquel Creek. Ahead was a little house under trees.

"Woah!" panted Travis. "Ever read *The Lord Of The Rings?*"

"Three times," puffed Brandon, scanning around. "This is like the Wythewindle Valley when the Hobbits started out on their quest."

"Just don't go to sleep under Old Man Willow. He's waiting right over there."

The little house was ancient and shabby, nestled along the edge of the stream and overshadowed by huge willow trees; nothing more than a ramshackle cottage that might have once been painted green. Behind it was a big wooden shed, buried in ivy and blackberry vines. Its rough old boards had never known paint and were weathered to rat-colored gray. Part of it boasted a second story with a mossy water tank on its roof. A windmill circled lazily in a salt-scented breeze from the ocean, which lay half a mile down the creek.

The house's front yard was a jungle of flowers, the kind that were usually treated like weeds, and just large enough for the Volkswagen van between the hillside and the creek. The dwelling was heavily decorated with everything from old street signs -- Speed Limit, Stop, and Railroad Crossing -- to hubcaps and grimacing tiki gods. Other gods had been carved from logs and glowered from under veils of ivy like refuges from Easter Island. Many old long-boards lay here and there in various stages of decomposition as if they'd come here to peacefully die. Squirrel and bird-feeders hung from trees, and smoke drifted up from a rusty stovepipe.

"Boss," said Brandon.

Travis chuckled. "I think we've entered another dimension. Or maybe we finally got *there*."

Ivy shrouded the house's front porch and fountained up through cracks in the boards. A scowling row of little uglies squatted along the vine-covered rail and seemed to be warning intruders away. An enormous armchair stood by the door and somehow looked like an ancient throne. A ratty old sofa was sagging beside it, and empty beer bottles lay everywhere; mostly Budweisers, Brandon noted, as he and Travis approached the steps.

"What's that smell?" asked Travis. "Besides breakfast cooking?"

"Fiberglass," said Brandon. "Resin for making surfboards."

The house's front windows, tall and narrow, were frosted with decades of grime. The door was open except for the screen, and the scent of bacon and eggs wafted out. A driftwood plank was nailed to the wall and carved with the words, TIKI ISLAND. The sound of a radio came from within, the end of the Beach Boys' *Surfer Girl* song, and there followed a rapid-fire DJ's voice:

"K.M.B.Y., 1240, Monterey. Home of the boss jocks!"

"Never heard that station," said Travis. "I checked 'em all out when we moved here."

"It's AM," said Brandon. "Or was. I didn't think it was still on the air. Mom said it used to be rock, but that was back in the 1960s."

Travis regarded the sagging steps. "Think the porch will hold me? …That's something else you should know, I have to watch for stuff like that... and breaking chairs and couches."

"Well, it's old but it still looks strong. Lean on my shoulder, I'll help you up."

A cow bell hung from a rope near the door, and Brandon clattered it gently after helping Travis climb to the porch. There came the sound of slow, heavy steps creaking across an ancient floor, and Brandon thought of first meeting Ro. Then a figure appeared in the shadows behind the rusty screen.

...And kept on appearing!

Brandon drew back in amazement, bumping into Travis's belly

218

and sinking in a little. The man in the doorway was huge beyond huge. He was roll upon roll of golden-brown fat, and maybe, thought Brandon, Hawaiian. He was wearing nothing that Brandon could see except for a shark-tooth necklace between the enormous orbs of his chest. His eyes were as black as the space between stars, and his ebony hair was an avalanche that cascaded over his shoulders. One mighty hand held a spatula, and he puffed an Italian cigar. Brandon couldn't guess his age: his face looked youthful despite triple chins, but he might have been twenty or fifty. He cheerfully grinned at the awe-stricken boys, obviously used to their reaction.

"Maybe a thousand," he said. "But who's counting."

"Um?" asked Travis. "How did you know I was wondering that?"

"Logical progression of thought."

"I shouldn't have worried about the porch."

"You're safe, it's under a spell." The huge man laughed. "But I won't tempt the tikis by joining you. I'm Kimo. And you guys are Travvy and Brandy. Bosco said you were coming."

"Hi," said Brandon, trying not to stare at the man, who made even Travis look small.

"Bocso's still up in his room," said Kimo. "Friday night, you know how that is." He pointed with the spatula to the ivy-covered shed. "Tell him breakfast is just about ready."

Leaving his board on the porch, Brandon helped Travis descend the steps and they went around the little house on a narrow path through waist-high flowers. One of the shed's double doors was open, revealing a dirt-floored surfboard shop. Rough wooden workbenches lined the walls, and long-boards stood or lay everywhere, as well as filling the rafters above. One was obviously just being built the way they'd been made in another time with redwood stringers and shiny brass screws, while others were undergoing repair. There were also lots of Tikis who seemed to be supervising the work. Sawdust covered the floor, while cans of paint and fiberglass resin were crammed on sagging shelves. A Volkswagen engine was being rebuilt... as far as Brandon could tell.

Beer seemed to be the primary fuel that powered this primitive factory, judging from all the empties. Sunlight shafted through cracks in the walls wherever the blackberries hadn't invaded, and dust motes danced in the golden beams. Water trickled down from above with a soothing liquid musical sound, and the windmill creaked with a sleepy rhythm.

Travis pointed. "I guess that's a real owl up there?"

Brandon peered up at the shadowy rafters. "Yeah, and I hope it stays up there."

At one side of the room was a steep, narrow staircase. A childish-looking sign said

TOLA RAT CLUBHOUSE
MEMBERS ONLY ⬆

and there was an arrow pointing up. Travis went over and paused at the foot, regarding the ancient board treads. "I don't think it's safe for me."

"I'm sure it's interracial," said Brandon.

"Funny, but you know what I mean."

"Maybe it's under a spell, too."

"For me that's tempting the tikis."

"But you have to want to see Bosco's room; you know it's gotta be boss as beans."

"Sure I do, but..."

"*Déjà vu*," said Brandon. "Can we do it? Sure we can."

"Are you always this mookin' optimistic?"

"Are you always this mookin' pessimistic?"

"This isn't gonna be easy," said Travis. "This thing's a lot steeper than my stairs at home and there's no banister to grab: you're gonna have to help with my belly, lift and push it out of the way so I can get my knees up."

"Let's do this," said Brandon.

Every tread groaned under Travis's weight and sagged way down in the middle while Brandon wrestled with Travis's blubber. Finally, panting and pouring sweat, Travis reached the top of the stairs and Brandon had to nudge him aside because he just stood there in evident awe.

The room was about twenty feet square, and vines had invaded through cracks in the walls. The windows were heavily crusted with dust, the sun streaming warm and golden through one and glowing leaf-green through another. The walls were papered with pictures and posters of beaches and surf scenes, and there were cartoons that featured Rat Fink.

The place was in absolute primal chaos as if the Big Bang had just occurred, and seemed to contain every possible thing that a boy could amass in fourteen years. There were comics, magazines, books and toys, model cars and monster figures... The Mummy, The Werewolf, and Frankenstein. There were little bottles of Testors paints, plus all the boxes the stuff had come in. There were green Army men, a brown teddy bear, a sea shell collection, dried starfish, an Erector set and a big tool box.

Two tables served as a desk and workbench. Another skateboard was being born from a wooden plank and steel wheels, and this one had a primitive tail. A tiki sat on its own little throne with a candle flickering at its feet. A crate was filled with actual records and there was a "Hi-Fi" to play them on. Another crate held a few clothes, mostly jeans and T-shirts; and the only shoes in sight were the battered old U.S. Keds. Beer cans and bottles lay everywhere, along with a million candy bar wrappers... Milky Way, Snickers and Three Musketeers. There were lots of potato chip bags, and a tuna can full of cigar butts. Water dripped from the ceiling, probably from the tank overhead, and two rusty buckets were placed to catch it.

"Hate to say it," said Brandon. "But this even blows away your bitchin' crib."

"Hear me arguing?" said Travis. "What's that thing over there on the table? Looks like a space ship radio from the Buck Rogers era."

"I think it's an eight-track player... or maybe a four-track like in Bosco's van."

Bocso lay naked asleep on his bed, which was nothing more than a shabby old mattress thrown on a frame of two-by-fours with a couple of olive-drab Army blankets. His tangled mop of bushy blond hair totally covered his eyes, and the cartoon rat seemed to glow on his shoulder as if it had been newly drawn.

It came to Brandon what Tommy had meant about being attracted to Bosco in a way that was hard to explain. It wasn't just his cute chubbiness that seemed to invite a teddy-bear hug, if not an actual cuddle; he was... well, the perfect boyhood friend who could always sleep over without any plans and would sooner die than break a promise; who always lived on the wrong side of town, always had matches, a sharp pocketknife, and often beer on his breath. He never seemed to take showers, but smelled more earthy and wild than bad, and totally lost his shirt all summer. He chewed with his mouth open, blasted burps, clutched his fork like a little kid, and made Satan blush in hell when he cursed. He pissed anywhere he had to go -- including your back yard -- never felt shy about jacking-off any time of day or night, and knew every dirty joke in the world... and could explain them if necessary. He could sneak into any movie theater, pet the meanest junkyard dog, spit on your cut and make it all better, and always made your parents nervous.

"No mirror," said Brandon.

"Zot?" said Travis.

"Tommy said he wouldn't have a mirror."

"'Cause he's never been taught he needed one."

"Very perceptive."

Travis shrugged. "The other logical explanation: it wouldn't show his reflection."

Brandon moved to wake Bosco: he could have called but wanted to touch him, maybe to confirm he was real. but Travis held him back.

"Check this out." Travis bent down laboriously and snagged an empty beer can. "This thing is steel, no pop-top either."

"We have one of those openers," said Brandon. "It's in a kitchen drawer somewhere."

"And when was the last time you used it?"

"I've seen those cans in antique stores. Most of them haven't been opened 'cause it makes 'em more collectable." Brandon scanned around again. "They have lots of things like what's in here... like these forty-five records and Muntz four-track tapes."

222

Travis held the can to his nose. "Smells fresh as yesterday to me. How long does beer stay good in a can?"

"I never kept any for more than a day."

"And who'd drink beer that was sixty years old, give or take a decade or two?"

"What are you saying?" asked Brandon.

"Lets do The Time Warp again."

"C'mon, man, you don't *really* think...?"

"I think I could, really easy."

Brandon knelt beside a box. "He's got some cool books... *Huckleberry Finn, Treasure Island, Swiss Family Robinson, Robinson Crusoe*... no relation."

"Pardon my duh," said Travis.

"*Kidnapped, Alice In Wonderland, The Wind In The Willows, The Jungle Book, Kim*. I've read all these. Have you?"

"Fat kids have tons of time to read."

"Here's *Lord Of The Rings* and *The Hobbit, Space Cadet* and *War Of The Worlds*..."

"He's probably got *The Time Machine*, too." Travis scanned around again. "Where's his surfing poster?"

"Huh?"

"Like the one you have on your wall."

"Troy made that for me." Brandon glanced at Bosco again. "They probably didn't do one of him, 'cause..."

"Yeah, 'cause he's fat," said Travis. "But where's the magazine cover at least? Dude wins something cool like that... the coolest summer he had in his life... you'd think he'd want to remember it. He'd have a whole bunch of those magazines. These are totally ancient. Check out the covers... kids on long-boards."

"I don't think he cared about winning. ...In fact, I'd guess he was seduced into entering."

"Interesting choice of words."

"Tommy can explain it."

"Or maybe it hasn't happened yet." Travis waved a hand. "Like this is some kind of loop in time that just keeps going round and round like an eight-track tape."

"Or in this case a four-track," said Brandon. "And we should put that in our story."

"Assuming we can get out of the story before we get caught in the loop."

"Hi, dudes." Bosco rolled onto his back. Like most boys his age he woke hard, but innocently wasn't shy about it. He pushed the hair out of his eyes, and yawned and stretched like a puppy.

"Guess I overslept again." He glanced at a clock that sat on a box... one of those clocks with bells on top, the kind you saw in old cartoons. "Guess I forgot to wind it. Heh. Friday night, you know how that is." He flicked a bit of potato chip from one of his innie nipples. "You guys know what time it is?"

"I'd say about 1963," said Travis, looking around again.

"That was a good year, Travvy." Rolling from the bed, his shaft poking out below his belly as if pointing the way, Bosco padded to one of the buckets to splash his face and a lot of the floor. "'Cept for what happened to President Kennedy."

"That won't happen for two more months. Maybe we should call the White House and warn him not to go to Dallas."

Bosco shrugged. "If you were old would you listen to us?"

Brandon said, "Maybe we did and they didn't."

Travis turned to Bosco. "Your dad said breakfast was just about ready."

"Bitchin'," said Bosco. "But Kimo ain't my real dad, he adopted me. My parents got drowned when I was a baby. We were out on a cruise an' the boat hit a rock. Happened off Molokai, but I was in a basket an' got washed up on a beach."

"Oh, sorry, man," said Brandon. "I mean about your 'rents."

"Thanks, but it was a long time ago." Bosco put on his cutoffs, stuffing in his mischievous shaft and buttoning them half way. "Hope you dudes are hungry. I told Kimo you were comin' so he probably cooked a ton. Then we'll do them surfin' lessons. Both you guys'll be up like magic."

"I almost believe that," said Travis.

"I didn't bring my board," said Brandon. "We rode the bus to Capitola and they don't let boards on the bus."

"That's okay," said Bosco. "It's better to learn on the regular kind. I got one that's perfect for you." He smiled his beaver smile at Travis. "An' another one perfect for you."

"Quadruple XL, I hope," said Travis.

"It was Kimo's when he was a kid."

"So, he's always been fat?" asked Travis.

"Ever since I known him, an' that seems like forever."

"Could be." Travis went to one of the tables to study what looked like a huge radio. "Is this how you contact the mother ship?"

"Nah, that's a NAB cartridge player like radio stations use. Found it at the dump… people throw tons of cool stuff away." Bosco came over and flipped a switch, then popped in a tape and flipped more switches. Dials lit up and gauge needles quivered. Big old speakers began to hum. Then a DJ's voice crackled out:

"*K.M.B.Y., 1240. Monterey. Home of the boss jocks!*"

There was a clatter of teletype sounds, then: "*In the news today, Soviet Premier, Nikita Khrushchev, called upon all the peace-loving nations to stand against U.S. imperialist aggression and its secret plan for world-domination. …There's a laugh and a half! …And now for the IMPORTANT news! Weather around the Big Bay today is sun and surf for everybody, with temperatures into the high 70s. …Now, here's a new sound by the Beatles, 'She Loves You,' yeah, yeah, YEAH!*"

"…Oh," said Brandon. "I guess there's another one in your house?"

"Yeah," said Bosco.

"What's this?" asked Travis, pointing to small wooden box. It had straps like a backpack, and there was a set of headphones attached that might have come from an ancient airplane.

"Made that," said Bosco. "To listen to tunes when I skate. There's a four-track player inside, an' a motorcycle battery. You strap it on your back an' listen through the headphones, an' it only weighs about twenty pounds."

"That's a boss idea," said Travis. "You oughta give Sony a call."

Brandon was listening to the "new" Beatles sound. "Wasn't that the beginning of the end for surf music?"

"Nah, dude," said Bosco. "Surf never dies."

TWENTY-FOUR

Breakfast was magically delicious with eggs, bacon, fluffy pancakes, glasses of milk and orange juice, plus rich Hawaiian Kona coffee. The Big Kahuna *was* wearing something besides his shark tooth necklace; a yellow sarong with a flowered pattern, though it couldn't be seen in a frontal view. Wetsuits were found for Travis and Brandon, pulled from a talcum-powdered pile that filled a living room corner, and every suit was old-fashioned black.

"I never would have believed it," said Travis, as Bosco zipped him up. "This actually fits!"

"I'll rub some wax on the zipper," said Bosco, snagging a candle from a tiki's shrine. "It's kinda stiff from layin' around, an' you'll probably wanna unzip it again. They get really hot when you're not in the water."

Brandon zipped his own well-fitting suit, which might have belonged to a slimmer Bosco; maybe before he'd chubbed-up this past summer. "Hard to tell you're wearing it, though. 'Cause you're a big black Kahuna."

Kimo smiled. "That was mine when I was his age. Never throw anything away. The minute you do you'll need it again."

"So, you were as fat as me?" asked Travis.

Kimo laughed. "Never threw that away either. I'll go out and wake up the boards."

"I'll start the 'dub," said Bosco. "We gotta make two trips up the hill. I'll take The Big Kahuna first. Thirty-six horses ain't enough ponies to get us all up there at once."

Brandon turned to Travis after Bosco and Kimo left. "You have to

227

go?"

"I'm just fat, I don't suck my thumb."

"Just don't be shy about telling me. Or anything else you need."

"I feel like I'm giving you payback for slavery."

"Don't be a dork."

They went out onto the vine-covered porch, watching as Bosco loaded the boards and tied them on the Volkswagen's roof. "That must be yours," said Brandon, as Bosco hoisted a huge green monster striped with yellow lightning bolts.

"And that must be Kimo's," said Travis. "Looks more like a barge than a surfboard."

"I think the really ancient ones had coffin-noses like that."

"Strangely appropriate maybe."

Kimo climbed in through the double side doors and settled into a big armchair like a mighty brown king on a throne. The little van lowered noticeably and the tires flattened a bit. Lunch had been packed in a rusty cooler, and Bosco loaded another cooler filled with Budweiser longnecks. Then he got behind the wheel and the van clattered off in a cloud of blue smoke, chugging slowly up the slope.

"Might as well sit down," said Brandon. "At that speed it could take a while."

Travis studied the sagging sofa. "I have to be careful about what I sit on."

"I'm just skinny, not stupid; you told me that already. The chair looks plenty strong enough."

"But it's obviously Kimo's." Travis eyed the row of tikis glowering along the rail. "And they might not like me in his chair."

"You're wearing his wetsuit and they haven't attacked."

Travis carefully lowered his bulk. "Bosco was right about this suit, feels like a sauna in here."

"Peel it down to your waist. ...Here, I'll help."

Travis gazed out through the curtain of ivy as Brandon bared his midnight mass. "I could live in a place like this. They never even locked the door."

"They're standing guard," said Brandon, pointing to the tikis. He stripped his own suit down to his waist, then studied the peaceful creek-bank scene. It was hard to believe that a mile away was a bustling mall and a thousand people. "Be cool if this house was on a beach. If you were a writer you could live anywhere."

"A successful writer," said Travis. "And success always translates to money. Like, Mr. Akida's books are boss, but he still has to teach at that suckhole school."

Brandon watched the birds and squirrels having their breakfasts from various feeders. "You'd only need a computer."

"And therefore electricity."

"You could have a generator, like wind or water powered. Or a solar charger."

"Like a high-tech Robinson Crusoe."

Brandon smiled. "I could be your boy Friday."

"That *would* be payback for slavery."

Brandon sat down on the arm of the chair. "Ever have a girl-friend?"

"Interesting segue. How do you know I don't have one now?"

"Sorry, man. ...But I didn't think it was 'cause you were fat."

"I know you didn't," said Travis. "'Cause you don't think that way."

"What do you mean?" asked Brandon.

"No offense, but you're kind of innocent: it never seems to occur to you that I can't do everything you can... and don't apologize, 'cause it makes you a better person."

"Better than who? Or would that be whom?"

"Better than people who think they know what I can't do."

"Like, people who say you can't be happy?"

"And the ones who won't let me. The self-appointed experts who say I can't be happy... while doing everything they can to make damn sure I can't."

"Yeah," agreed Brandon. "People who think they know what's best have probably mooked up more people's lives than all the haters in the world."

"I had a girlfriend in Oaktown," said Travis. "And she wasn't an admirer or a chubby chaser."

"I didn't even think that."

"Sorry, I keep forgetting you're you." Travis smiled again. "I won't say she didn't like my fat... I cuddle really good... but she was deeper than that."

"She'd have to be deep for you to like her. ...Think you'll see her again?"

"Probably not. We messaged for awhile, but it's not the same as being there."

"I'm sure you'll meet somebody else."

"It's gonna take somebody special."

"'Course it will," said Brandon, "And I'm not being politically-correct. Like, sure, she'll have to be smart and cool, but I'm not pretending you're not fat."

"Don't forget the sex."

"...I did."

"But she might not."

"I didn't think of that."

"I can still be a father, it just won't be as much fun getting there... either for me or her."

"...I think I know what you mean. And you'd make a real good father."

"How would you know?"

"Ro, duh, you're the man to him."

"Thanks, but don't forget my dad, he's been the man for both of us. ...You ever have a girlfriend?"

Brandon shrugged. "I was too stoned to care last year. Maybe the time when I should have been caring and learning how to play the game. And now it's like I'm still waking up."

"Your eyes are open, what do you see?"

"That I wasted a year of my life. Year thirteen, up in smoke. A year I don't remember much, and a year I can never live over again. I haven't been learning to run the race. The race to be cool, or get a girl, or... I dunno, to be a 'success,' whatever the mook that means."

"Maybe you don't have to learn."

"Because I'm white and my 'rents have money?"

"How much truth can you take?"

"All I can get, which hasn't been much."

Travis thought for a moment. "When you're black you waste a lot of time thinking about being black. Like, what you should be able to do, but what you probably can't do... or what's gonna be a lot harder for you." Travis patted his belly. "In a way it's like being born this fat, except it's weight you can never lose. When do you think about being white?"

"A lot since I met you."

"My bad," said Travis.

"Your good," said Brandon, "because it's true. I *don't* have to try as hard as you, and I never learned survival skills... not the kind you've had to learn."

"Your 'rents are survivors, learn from them."

"They used to be survivors," said Brandon. "But now they're just good at running the race. Commuting over the hill every day... leave in the dark, come home in the dark. No time to kick back and do what they want. ...But what's the prize they're running for?"

"Maybe where they live right now. And all the things they have."

"But they don't have *time* to enjoy those things, so what's the point of having them?" Brandon gazed out at the flowers and trees. "Some-times I think they forgot what they wanted. What they *really* wanted, I mean. Or else they pretend it wasn't important. Like a phase they just think they grew out of."

"I'd say you've learned a lot," said Travis. "Maybe you just don't know it yet 'cause you haven't had to use it."

TWENTY-FIVE

The van rolled north on Highway One, leaving Santa Cruz behind where vallies were swarming over the hill to blanket the beaches and bustle the Boardwalk and scent the air with tanning oil. There wasn't much room on the narrow front seat, and Brandon was almost buried in fat, immobilized between Travis's mass and Bosco's rolly baby-chub. 36 horses were earning their oats, push-ing Kimo's enormous weight, along with Travis's 500 pounds. Added to that were Bosco and Brandon, the four long-boards and the cooler of beer. The Volkswagon managed to reach 55, but only after a takeoff run after leaving Mission Street that seemed to go on forever. They clattered along the rugged coast where fields were planted with brussel sprouts and spiky rows of artichokes between the road and the edge of the cliffs that overlooked the sea. The Surfaris sang on the four-track deck above the engine's rattling beat, and the sun was hot and bright in the sky. The boys had their suits peeled down to their waists, and the air inside the little van was a stew of sweat and neoprene, and smogged with strong tobacco smoke.

"You okay, Brandon?" asked Travis.

"Yeah," said Brandon, trying to breathe. A ton of Travis lay on his leg and was slowly putting it to sleep. He sucked a hit off the nasty cigar, coughed, and passed it back to Bosco. "*That's* ten years off my life for sure."

Bosco laughed, his chest overlapping the steering wheel. "But that's at the end of your life, dude, which is usually skeezy anyhow." He thrust his hand between Brandon's legs to grasp the gear shift lever. "Nothin' personal, heh."

232

"Third is cool," said Brandon. "It's fourth that gets kinda personal."

Their speed dropped down to about 35 as they chugged up yet another hill. The engine sounded like Tommy's mower, though maybe not as powerful. Brandon turned to Travis and pointed. "Down there's the Free Beach I told you about."

Bosco blew out smoke. "All beaches should be free."

"No offense, Brandy," said Kimo, kicked on his throne behind the boys. "But white people love doing that kind of stuff. Wherever there's anything nice in the world they fence it in and put up signs and make you pay to see it. That really pisses off the tikis."

Brandon smiled. "The Free Beach is where you go naked."

"You a nudie?" asked Bosco.

"Nah, anybody can go there."

"Even girls?"

"Yeah. But I was too young to appreciate that the last time I was there." Brandon laughed. "But, Chad sure did; and it's hard to hide your feelings when there's nothing to hide 'em under."

Travis chuckled. "I don't have that problem. Do fat kids go there, too?"

"I don't remember seeing many; the place is kind of New Age and old hippe and their kids are always skinny, but sometimes we took Tommy and all the kids wanted to play with him."

Travis smiled. "Most little kids are attracted to fat ones. Like, it's instinctive or something. They come up to Ro all the time at the beach and wanna feel his blubber. Sometimes their parents get freaked; here's these white kids hanging with Ro and looking like they're worshipping him. Some of 'em stick out their tummies. One little dude came back to play with a beachball under his shirt."

"That's called stuffing," said Brandon. "Tommy said when little kids stuff it could be a sign of future gainers."

Kimo said, "I don't know about 'stuff' like that. But little kids being attracted to fat *is* normal and instinctive. Fat means you're healthy and going to live. It's the runt of the litter, the skinny one, who may not survive. Kids have to be taught to hate fat kids like they have to be taught to hate anything."

233

"But in nature, if you got really fat you couldn't hunt."

"As far as nature's concerned, if you're really fat, you don't need to hunt."

"But, what about running away?" asked Brandon. "Like, from lions and tigers and bears?"

"In a natural fat scenario, the lions and tigers and bears would be fat."

That put a picture in Brandon's mind of a lion whose belly was dragging the ground, waddling after a fat antelope in a comical slow-motion chase.

Kimo added, "Not all people had predators they had to run away from. The Pacific Islands had many cultures where food was naturally plentiful and being fat was beautiful."

"Some parts of Africa, too," said Travis. "A lot of cultures think fat kids are cool."

"It's totally boss in Hawaii," said Bosco. "Lots of Hawaiian kids are fat."

"Were you raised in Hawaii?" asked Brandon?

"As much as I can remember."

"In a little grass shack?" asked Travis.

"Nah, just the regular kind of shack. Kimo was a grave-digger. We lived in a graveyard close to the beach."

Travis murmured to Brandon, "'Raised' makes a pun, you notice. Bosco... graveyard...?"

"It also makes a cool story." Brandon looked out the window. "Where are we going, Bosco? We'll be in Davenport soon."

"North of there," said Bosco.

"I didn't know there were any surf beaches between Santa Cruz and Half Moon Bay. Except Pescadero."

"It's a secret," said Bosco, shifting up to fourth again as the van topped yet another hill. "If you tell anybody the tikis will get ya."

The van rattled on up the coast, slowed to a crawl on the up-grades but rocketing down the opposite slopes. They climbed again into more rolling hills. Above the cliffs overlooking the sea were fields of yellow-green brussel sprouts. Bosco slowed down and swung off the highway. They jolted along a narrow dirt road, splashed through several lakes of mud, and finally stopped at a padlocked gate. There was a sign: NO TRESPASSING.

"Here's a beach with a sign and a fence," said Travis.

"It's 'cause of the sprouts," said Bosco. He took a key from the ashtray.

Brandon made a face. "Who'd wanna steal brussel sprouts?"

"They ain't too bad with butter."

"Old friends of my family's," said Kimo, as Bosco got out to unlock the gate. "Japanese-Americans. They almost lost this land during World War Two. They were sent to an internment camp for the crime of looking different."

"I read about that," said Travis. "Their Constitutional rights were taken away by the government because they were considered a 'threat.'"

"Yeah," said Brandon. "A lot of them did lose their property. And their stores and houses."

"My father worked for them," said Kimo. "Took care of this place until after the war so the government couldn't take it." He pointed. "The Army used to have guns on those cliffs. In case of submarines, I guess; but any fool should have seen the reefs and known they couldn't have come in close."

Bosco opened the gate, drove the van through and re-locked the gate behind them. The trail grew muddier crossing the fields, and they wallowed and rocked over ruts and holes, and splashed through more glimmering puddles. Finally, they came to the edge of the cliffs and there was a little cove below.

"Here she is, dudes," said Bosco. "Ain't Molokai but she's good for practice. ...See where they curl on the reefs out there? Gives you a totally bitchin' ride! Almost a whole quarter-mile."

"Um," said Brandon. "Those waves look kinda big."

"More than kinda," said Travis.

"Nah, dudes, that ain't big. Wait till the tide goes out. *Then* they get big."

"...Oh," said Brandon.

"I feel kinda small," said Travis. "Which normally isn't my thing."

"How do we get down there?" asked Brandon.

"And back up again?" added Travis. "No way I could walk it."

"No sweat, Travvy," said Bosco. "There's sort of a road, but we gotta unload some weight again. These brakes ain't the best. I'm gonna reline 'em next week. I'll take the Big Kahuna first an' then come back for you guys."

Travis and Brandon got out, and the van clattered off trailing smoke. They watched it descend a narrow trail that was probably made for Army jeeps.

"I'm way too fat to be here," said Travis.

Brandon laughed. "*Déjà vu* again."

"I'm serious, man." Travis faced the sea. "Way too fat and way too small."

Brandon gazed out at the towering waves, which broke in ranks to thunder ashore. There were line after line of emerald green, each wave topped with a snowy crown, rising, rolling, rushing in, flinging up clouds of silver spray that drifted over the cliffs. They would make a bitchin' ride, he thought... unless, of course, he wiped-out.

"This is probably a mistake," said Travis.

"I'm scared, too," said Brandon. "If it makes you feel any better."

"Is it supposed to?"

"I was scared of your feast the first night I met you. Does that put anything into perspective?"

"Why?"

"I thought I'd look uncool."

"Why?"

"I thought I couldn't eat a lot. Like, I'd be insulting you and your 'rents."

Travis smiled. "I'm touched. But sometimes people get killed for cool. How cool is that?"

"I trust Bosco. Don't you?"

"I think I do, but I don't know why."

"So, if he says we're ready for this, then I guess we are."

"Because I got up in your swimming pool?"

"You can't sink in a wetsuit. That's why scuba divers need weights. And *you* couldn't sink if you wanted to."

"Ever wonder how Bosco drowned?"

"Oh, shut up. ...Listen, man, if you lose your board just keep your cool... and you've got tons of that. The waves will carry you back to the beach. If a wave breaks over you, hold your breath. It'll seem like forever but it's not very long, maybe half a minute."

"I'll try to remember that when I panic." Travis laughed. "It's easy for Bosco. Like, what's he got to be scared of? ...Assuming he's already dead? Maybe he wants us to join him where it's always Endless Summer 1963."

"C'mon, man," said Brandon. "You don't *really* think...?"

Travis regarded the ocean. "I don't know what to think anymore after seeing his room. The dude is decades out of date, along with everything he has and just about all he seems to know. He doesn't buy stuff, he makes his own. He invents things that are already invented. He listens to a radio station that doesn't exist anymore. ...Civil Rights are only a dream. John F. Kennedy is President. And kids are doing the Twist."

"Invented by Chubby Checker, a black dude."

"It's cool you know black history. But, Bosco was raised in a grave-yard... 'raised' one way or another... by a dude who believes in tiki gods. After being washed up on a beach. What would you think?"

"You have a boss imagination, and we'll get an A on our story."

"Our book, you mean," said Travis. "That's what it's turning into."

"Well," said Brandon. "Assuming Bosco isn't a ghost, are you saying he should try to be cool... what other people think is cool... start buying and consuming things... maybe starting with a mirror... lose some weight and get in the race?"

"Assuming he isn't a ghost," said Travis. "Or a time surfer, or someone from a parallel universe or an alternate dimension... which has yet to be decided, I don't think he'd do that. Like he said at your party, he's the star of his own life. ...Or maybe his afterlife."

"We were assuming he isn't a ghost, or any of the other possibles."

"Whatever he is, he doesn't belong in this time and place when everybody is trying to be the kind of stars they're told to be. ...And assuming he *is* somebody who surfed through time, or jumped from one time into another on one of his homemade skates or boards, he's either gotta be from the past or the alternate future that should have happened. Again, he doesn't belong in *this* time... this time, or alternate universe, can't tolerate people like him. Maybe he's even a threat to it, like he brought something here it can't deal with... maybe a kind of Endless Summer; the summer from 1963 that *should* have happened for everybody."

Brandon smiled. "Maybe for him that's 42... if we want to believe it. And maybe that's why there are always some people who never seem to belong in a time; who either seem behind the time or maybe way ahead of the time."

Travis nodded. "This time has to really hate people like him, 'cause they show other people how mooked it is."

"We gotta put that in our story."

"Which brings us back to this time," said Travis, turning toward the sea to watch the crashing waves.

Brandon touched his shoulder. "You don't have to surf. We're on a boss beach, it's a bitchin' day. You could kick in the sand, drink beer and enjoy it."

"But, it would be so uncool if I didn't." Travis shook his head. "Here's a dude who weighs five-hundred pounds and he's worried about looking uncool."

"You're a quarter-ton of cool."

Travis looked around at the fields, the gentle, girlish hills to the east, golden brown in the Indian Summer heat and dotted with groves of green oak trees beneath a clear blue sky. Then he turned west toward the shimmering sea.

"Describe the scene," said Brandon. "Like you were writing a story."

"A whole different planet... or maybe a time."

"That's not a very descriptive picture."

"I'm totally out of my picture," said Travis. "Four months ago my world was a block. As far as I could manage to waddle down to the corner market, unless I took a bus somewhere. But now I can see for miles, and that's a little scary when you've never seen that far before." He shrugged. "But, we're here now, wherever here is, which

238

almost feels like halfway *there*. ...I think I need to piss."

Brandon laughed. "I'm your boy Friday in this time. Here, let me get you unzipped. ...Um, I guess Ro is... challenged, too? ...At least in that way, I mean."

"If he's outside and has to go he can rest his belly on something," said Travis as Brandon unzipped his suit. "Like that big rock over there."

"...Couldn't you?"

"Sure."

"Then why am I holding yours? ...And why did I do it this morning? You could have used the bank by the road going down to Bosco's."

"Sure," said Travis again.

"...You're always testing me, aren't you? ...Like on the first day of school; you *knew* you couldn't reach your pack when you put it on the floor. You wanted to see if I'd get it for you. ...Why? Because I might have been a hater and wanted to make you suffer?"

"Maybe I'm writing another book; The Adventures Of A Quarter-ton Kid."

"Are you?"

"I'm writing in my mind right now."

"Gonna put me in it?"

Travis laughed. "You're already in it. ...Now you can zip me up again."

"How do you manage in school?" asked Brandon.

"I don't drink a lot so I won't have to go. If I do, I have to sit down."

"In the handicapped stall?"

"Not if I can help it, in case a handicapped dude needs it."

"I could help," said Brandon. "And it's not payback for slavery."

"Wanna get assigned as my aide? Like that dude who helps that dude who's in a wheelchair?"

"He's pretty fat, too."

"He's fat 'cause he's in a wheelchair, he's not in a wheelchair 'cause he's fat." Travis looked down at himself as Brandon zipped his suit. "That would be easy for me. Like, get so fat I really can't walk."

239

He smiled. "And meet somebody like you. Sometimes I even think about it."

Brandon laughed. "Like you said, you're just fat, you don't suck your thumb."

"Zot?"

"Another thing Tommy told me about; people wanting... or at least fantasizing... about getting so fat they're as helpless as babies and need someone to take care of them. A basic return to infancy when someone else totally cared for you."

"Sort of like never growing up and having to deal with life on your own."

"Sometimes growing up scares me."

"And no doubt there are people who want... or at least fantasize... about taking care of somebody that fat?"

"It's a big universe," said Brandon. "I guess there's room for every-thing. But, speaking hypothetically, I'd guess being in a wheelchair would stop a lot of the hate. At least people would think you got fat..."

"'Cause I was handicapped."

"Yeah."

"Which is why I don't, 'cause I'm not."

"Um," asked Brandon. "You could lose weight, couldn't you? I mean without drugs or getting cut open."

"Sure," said Travis. "But, being fat is who I am. I thought we established that. I've been fat for fourteen years, and there's too many things I wanna learn besides how to be a skinny dude." He patted Brandon's shoulder. "And I meet cool people like you who restore my faith in humanity."

Brandon smiled. "Thanks. But what about all the hate?"

"*Déjà vu* again: I'd be trading one kind of hate for another, 'cause that's the mooked-up time we're in."

"Which sure as mook feels like the wrong time that never should have happened." Brandon pulled up Travis's suit. "Wanna do another beast-feast? We could have it at my house. Maybe on Halloween night. My 'rents will go to their company party... I think they almost have to. They'll stay at some Silicon Valley hotel. And

240

Chad will be at another party. We could invite all the beasts."

"What about Jason?"

"Zot?"

"I feel kinda sorry for him."

"Sometimes so do I," said Brandon. "But, the dude needs professional help. I told you what happened on Thursday with Tommy in the ice cream shop."

"He does need help," agreed Travis. "But nobody *wants* to help him. He's just another 'obese' kid who nobody is supposed to like."

"But he's really hard to like."

"Which is what the haters want. ...But, are we not beasts?"

"So, you think I should ask him?"

Travis shrugged. "He might not want to come, but at least he'll know we don't hate him. Like, we left the Transporter on and he can beam up if he wants to."

"Okay," said Brandon. "And everybody could dress like on Beastworld. ...Or do you think that would be uncool? Like wearing stupid party hats?"

"Nah, it would be boss. Like a fat fur party."

The van came chugging up the trail. "Dudes!" called Bosco. "C'mon, hurry up, the tide's goin' out!"

Travis regarded the waves again. "Been bitchin' knowing you, Brandy-buck."

"Same here, Travvy-dude. ...Maybe we'll meet on other side where it's always Endless Summer."

"Why do I feel like I heard that before?"

"Maybe because we already have."

TWENTY-SIX

The four big long-boards went to sea like a surfing safari to some other time. Bosco was leading on Big Bertha Red; Brandon and Travis were following, while Kimo paddled along behind like a huge brown god watching over his godlets. Brandon had ridden Troy's board a few times at the sewer plant in Capitola, but a long-board was a whole different beast, sort of like riding Bosco's skate and having to learn all over again. Paddling it was hard, sweaty work, and his suit soon felt like a self-contained sauna. Travis was slow and clumsy at first until he found the right position and settled into a steady stroke.

The waves had looked huge from atop the cliffs, but here at eye-level they filled the sky. Yet they came roaring past in regular ranks instead of a random violence attack. This was perfect surfing surf, the kind real surfers would die to ride. It seemed strange they hadn't discovered this beach.

...Unless, thought Brandon, this place might *really* be somewhere else. Did Bosco surf through space and time as freely as he surfed the sea? And could he bring disciples along like Jonathan Livingston Seagull?

Brandon could almost believe that... especially now when his world was a board, a ten-foot plank of glistening gold with a fearfully grimacing tiki god who glowered defiance back at the waves.

Maybe these boards were just more buoyant than smaller modern models, but they always managed to crest the waves instead of your having to lie down flat and punch your way through a watery wall. Or maybe it was only good timing based on Bosco's experience? A quarter-mile was a long way to paddle, but finally they reached that peaceful place out beyond the breakers. The place where surfers told their tales. The place where nothing could catch them. The sun was warm in the clear blue sky, and the water sparkled emerald green.

"This is boss!" puffed Travis, slowly getting his breath back. "The land looks so different from way out here. It's like..."

Brandon smiled. "Long ago and far away?"

Kimo laughed. "That's the right perspective."

Bosco flipped the land a bird. "That's where all the skeezers live."

Kimo thumped his board with a fist. "Out here it's just you and the sea. And this is all you own." He smiled at Brandon, who was scoping around. "Don't worry about sharks." He fingered his necklace. "This keeps 'em away."

"Can you read my mind?" asked Brandon.

"A good observer can appear to read minds. You were at peace a minute ago, with yourself and the universe, but then you thought about sharks."

"It's like Lothlorien," said Bosco. "In *The Lord Of The Rings*. If there's bad stuff here you brought it with you."

Travis asked, "Kids used to read a lot, didn't they? Like, in 1963?"

"Yeah," said Kimo. "And they saw the world through their own eyes, and dreamed with their own imaginations instead of somebody else's. It's easier to watch a screen and someone else's view of the world than to imagine your own... the way you think it should look and be instead of what you're *told* it should be."

"And who you should hate?" asked Brandon.

"Brandy-buck wins a cigar. But this isn't a place to talk about hate."

"Or a time?" asked Travis.

"Time doesn't exist out here," said Kimo. "Not in the way you know it, Jim."

"It's time to catch a wave," said Bosco. "I'll pick us a totally boss one."

"Um," said Brandon. "I'd settle for one that was just slightly bitchin'."

"There's only one first-time, Brandy, so it's gotta be totally boss."

Kimo smiled. "This time's for you guys, I'll come in on the next one."

"In case we wipe out?" asked Travis.

Bosco laughed. "Them boards won't let you."

Travis looked down at his plank. "Somehow I almost believe that."

"Believing in something can help," said Kimo. "Especially if it's yourself."

Bosco pointed out to sea. "Here she comes! Kowabunga, dudes!"

"Pray for surf," said Brandon. He dug his hands into the water and paddled after Bosco.

"Somebody did," said Travis, and followed.

Brandon looked over his shoulder, seeing something being born, lifting its great green head from the sea. It seemed to shake itself from sleep and realize its awesome power.

Travis caught up. "Should I look?" he panted. "...I think I can see enough in your face."

"Keep your eyes on Bosco," said Brandon. "Do what he does when he does it."

"What if he jumps through a time warp?"

"Then we do the Time Warp again."

"I'm way too fat for this."

"Maybe this time you're just the right size."

Brandon could feel the pull of the wave, drawing him backward and into itself. He was rising fast, a scary feeling, an airplane caught in a mighty updraft being sucked into the sky. On another board he might have escaped by turning and paddling frantically back to that peaceful place beyond the breakers, but this board *wanted* to ride the wave! It was like a scarred old battle horse that only knew how to charge. It had never been taught to retreat.

Brandon wondered how old the board was, how many millions of waves it had ridden, how many bare feet had stood on its back, or even hung-ten on its puggy nose. This brave old board would despise his ass if he didn't stand up on his own two feet and ride it the way it was born to be ridden!

Behind him the wave was beginning to roar. Its lofty head was crowned with foam, rising, towering, filling the sky. This wave might have crossed the entire Pacific and now it was gathering all its strength to make that final rush to shore. It wanted a majestic death! And it wanted Brandon to honor that death by sharing the last of its life.

Brandon was lifted, higher, faster... he must have been above the cliffs. And still he seemed to be rising! This *couldn't* have been a wave from this time! Bosco must have called it up from when the sea had ruled the world!

He risked a look at Travis, whose ebony face was determined... just like in another time when he'd made a decision to walk down a hill and try to cross a little mud puddle. Travis smiled bravely and called, "Oh no, not again!"

The roar had risen to thunder, mounting louder every second until it battered Brandon's ears. His board was tilted steeply down, bucking like an angry horse when a timid rider fumbled the reins. Brandon quickly shifted his weight to bring its nose back up. Maybe he could still roll out, cut back over the curling crest and make the board abandon this ride?

And yet he knew, one way or another -- in shining triumph standing tall, or in disgrace and flat on his belly -- he had to make it to shore on his own.

His mind was a jumble of thoughts, and some were pretty cowardly... like escaping his fate by heading to sea and freezing out there like an eight-year-old grommet until the Coast Guard rescued him. ...Or, what if he paddled down the coast to slink ashore on a peaceful beach where puppy waves lapped at little kids' toes?

But there would be someone waiting for him; a boy with total disgust on his face. A boy who would never trust him again. A boy who would never like him again. ...A boy named Brandon Williams.

He was still gaining speed. The roar in his ears was deafening, the thunder of a thousand trains. The water around him was frothing white. He sucked a deep breath... it was time!

And then he was... UP!

And the board seemed to know it.

It shook itself like something freed, finding its rider worthy at last. Brandon balanced, spreading his arms. The downhill speed seemed to suck out his breath. His long hair streamed in the wind. Too fast! he thought. In seconds he might outrun the wave. Then it would catch him and smack him down! He shifted his stance, cutting sideways a little, almost amazed when the board obeyed.

Something huge and black shot past. Travis was up! His dreadlocks glistened with sliver spray. The lightning bolts on his board seemed to flash.

There was streak of raving red as Bosco cut between them, posed on the tips of five chubby toes, his other leg raised like dancer... a hood ornament on a classic car... the Coyote scanning for Roadrunners. Then he was gone in a swirl of spray.

Brandon rode on -- a clean quarter-mile -- learning the finer moves on the way. ...Or, was the board teaching him? He managed to get into Bosco's stance, even while cutting back and forth across the face of the watery wall. Then he crouched to enter the pipeline, that curling tunnel of glittering green that only a surfer could know.

Suddenly, there was the beach ahead, and the ride was over way too soon. Expertly now but feeling sad, he cut aside and pulled gracefully out. He couldn't have borne to ride the wave that last fifty feet to its death.

Travis shot past and also pulled out as if he'd been surfing all his life. "I guess this is sex in the ocean," he panted.

Bosco appeared in a haze of spray. "Them boards are yours. You just got married."

Kimo came cruising majestically in a tumbling welter of white. "Till death do you part."

TWENTY-SEVEN

The sound of surf echoed in Brandon's ears, eternally rolling and rushing in as each new wave was born to rise, to live its short life in roaring glory then die on the shore with a whisper. The sun was pleasantly hot on his chest as he lay with his back to a palm tree. The Free Mutant Boys had roasted an ox, and the meat had been basted with succulent sauce so its flavor was irresis-tible. They had eaten the whole mookin' thing! All were sprawled around the fire, and bones were scattered across the sand. Everyone else was asleep, even Panther-boy Kelvin, who should have been standing guard. He lay against a rock nearby, his six-pack belly as tight as a drum.

Brandon couldn't have gotten up if the Beastmaster's Army had landed. He lay in helpless ecstasy, his own belly bulging like a balloon swollen twice the size of Zach's, and what a bitchin' feeling!

"Open your mouth," pleaded Nikki. "Please! ...Oh. Bucky, I want you so bad!"

"I want you, too," moaned Brandon. He could hardly open his eyes anymore, but there she was bending over him, her beautiful breasts swinging free in the sun, brushing his glistening sauce-smeared chest as she tried to tempt him with even more food.

"Please, Bucky. Just one more bite and then we'll make love."

Brandon's alarm clock went off.

"Beans!" He punched the clock in its warbling face, sending it flying across the room, then lifted the sheet and peered underneath. "BEANS!"

"Brandon?" His mother's voice came from out in the hall. "Did you call me, honey?"

247

Brandon jerked the covers back up. "No, mom. I... just had a dream. ...How come you're still here?"

His mother opened the door. "We're just getting ready to leave. There was another wreck on the summit so we decided to wait a while. We'd just be part of a long parking lot if we'd tried to go over at six. I really hate that commute."

"Oh," said Brandon, hoping she wouldn't come over to kiss him. "Did you ever wish you could stop doing that and live on an island like you said?"

Darlene seemed to sigh. "I dream about that a lot these days. But that's life, running the race."

"Does it have to be?" asked Brandon.

"You'll understand when you're older."

"You don't have to do this for me."

Darlene looked puzzled. "Do what, honey?"

Brandon waved around. "Keep running the race to have all this stuff. I don't need it, mom. ...I mean, thanks, but..."

Darlene smiled. "Thank *you*, Brandon. You're really becoming a thoughtful young man since you... overcame your problem. But, I'm sure you'd feel differently somewhere else that wasn't as nice, and without all your things."

"I was happy on the Free Beach naked with you and dad and Chad."

"But what if it was cold or raining? Or we didn't have any food?"

"We'd survive. We'd build a shack out of driftwood and learn to fish and hunt. I used to think you were teaching us, me and Chad, how to survive."

Darlene laughed. "Did you? ...Well, maybe we would have survived. But life is more than survival, Brandon. People who only survive don't have time to enjoy their lives. Be thankful for the things you have, and don't feel guilty for having them. You didn't steal them from anyone."

"I didn't earn them either. And I didn't make any of them."

"You didn't have to earn your things. And you wouldn't know how to make anything."

Brandon gazed around. "Maybe that's part of the problem: we're

248

surrounded by things made with hate."

"...I don't understand," said Darlene.

"Hungry kids made a lot of these things. And most were made by poor people who can't afford to buy them. Those people have to hate what they're doing, and maybe who they're doing it for. So, all these things are full of hate. And we surround ourselves with them. Don't you think that hate leaks out?"

"That's an interesting concept, honey, but it's not realistic. Things are just things made of other things. Lifeless material possessions. Your father and I worked hard for our things, and so you and Chad could have them. I'm glad you feel compassion for others, and maybe a year in public school is a valuable lesson."

Brandon cocked his head. "What do you mean 'a year?'"

Darlene glanced at her watch. "I don't have time to discuss that now. Maybe at dinner tonight."

"If you make it home in time."

"I have to go, honey. Have a nice day." Darlene closed the door.

Brandon rolled out of bed. His hand was on the bathroom door-knob when he heard the shower start. "Wait a minute, I need to get in there!"

"Tough tit, dorkus," said Chad.

"C'mon, man!"

"If you gotta go, what's stopping you?"

"I need the shower, dammit!"

There was a two-second pause, then Chad broke into laughter. "Ooooo!"

"Shut up, dork!" yelled Brandon. He jerked the door open, getting a face full of Chad-scented steam. "Gimme a minute at least!"

Chad yanked open the shower curtain. "No way, twat, I'm running late." Then he laughed again. "Oh, that must have been a good one!"

"Bite me, Chad! Move your ass over and let me in there!"

"The mook I will! You're not getting close to me like that. And don't even think about using the sink until I'm done with shaving."

"Damn you, dork!"

"Use the guest bathroom, stupid."

"The tub's all full of junk!"

Chad rolled his eyes. "Oh, get your ass in here, dweeb! Four bathrooms in this big empty barn and I have to share this one with you."

"The feeling is mutual, butt-head!"

Chad laughed again. "I guess it wasn't intentional or you would have used a sock."

"Boy-genius wins a cigar."

"Was it good?"

"It could have been. Except for the mookin' clock going off."

"Don't you hate when that happens in the middle of sexual ecstasy?"

"Shut up and give me the soap."

"Do I want the graphic details? Paint me a porno picture with words."

"Why not," muttered Brandon, soaping himself. "A tropical island. Turquoise water, silver sand. A beach, the surf, the green palm trees..."

"And native girls? ...Bare-breasted of course?"

"Sure wasn't native boys."

"That's a relief. You haven't mentioned girls for a month."

"Doesn't mean I haven't been thinking about 'em."

"Try more manual methods."

"Apparently twice a day isn't enough."

Chad studied his brother. "Off-topic, wet one, but you're really starting to get a belly. Bet you can't even suck it flat."

"Who do I have to pose for? ...And, you haven't worked-out for a week. Troy's getting more ripped than you."

"I've been picking up Christine in the mornings. She lives in Rio Del Mar, so I don't have time."

"Yeah?" said Brandon, scrubbing himself. "What happened to Lisa? She dumped you, huh?"

"It was a mutual dis-attraction."

"Some dude with more muscles and fewer brains?"

"Thanks for the brains. She was pretty shallow."

"I kinda liked her."

"You have a thing for big-breasted Barbies."

"Breasted, yes, Barbies, no. You could get up earlier, or work-out in the evenings."

"I don't have time anymore. And muscles aren't me... or not all of me. At least I can talk to Christine without always having to lose my shirt and let her pet me like a dog."

"I've seen you kiss like one."

"As if you knew anything about kissing. ...Here I am discussing my life with a pot-bellied punk who still has wet dreams. ...How did you get so fat in a month?"

"Hey, I'm not fat. I'm just finally starting to fill out a little."

"Yeah. *Way* out. And sideways, too." Chad grabbed Brandon around the waist. "Check the love-handles, chubby."

"Help, I'm being molested."

"Seriously, Brandon, what's up with you? You catching obesity from Tommy?"

Brandon laughed. "Tommy won his fat war last week. His mom had to buy him all new jeans, and he's only gained a pound since then. And she's making him normal meals."

"So, how come he's not getting twice as fat?"

"His mom's not trying to starve him, so he doesn't have to compensate by eating everything he can. And he's skating to school every day again instead of taking the bus. Meets up with Ro and they skate together. Travis's parents got their rib shop, and Ro bought a board from the money he makes washing dishes after school. Tommy helped him pick it out."

"A strong one, I hope."

"Bosco added stringers."

"So, they all lived happily ever after. ...But, how come you're getting fat?"

"I'm not *that* fat."

"Yeah, jelly-belly? So, how come you have to lean way over to see what you're doing down there?"

Brandon studied himself. "Maybe a little too much beer."

"Five-hundred brands and you wanted them all."

"I'm only drinking one a day in alphabetical order."

251

"What about on weekends? All those beach parties with Bosco?"

"They're not beach parties, we surf."

"And always come home with beer on your breath."

"My grades are good."

"So I've noticed. And your teachers like you... except for Mr. Mortimer, and of course the Coach." Chad patted Brandon's head. "Disregarding the fact that a brain-dead zombie could graduate from Lowbrow High, I'm proud of you, son. Proud, proud, proud, proud. ...But you're not skating as much anymore since Bosco's been picking you up. Plus breakfast with Tommy and lunch with your friends. ...Your fat friends."

"I thought they had your seal of approval."

"With noted reservations. But remember what I said about lying down with dogs."

"Just because you hang with fat kids doesn't mean you have to get fat. There's no peer-pressure like hanging with druggies."

"That's not a convincing argument." Chad poked Brandon's belly. "In view of the weighty evidence. You're really getting chubby, man! Doesn't it hang over your jeans?"

"Not when I sag."

"There's only so low you can go, rolly-one. ...Have you really looked in a mirror lately? You're even getting boy-boobs."

"Nobody's making me eat," said Brandon.

"I've seen you having lunch with your gang; are any of them *losing* weight? Forget Travis, who you said has a problem. And a lot of Mexican dudes are fat. Same with Danny the Indian. But there's the dude with the basketball belly. And even that cute little kid you corrupted is starting to put on a pot."

"Rex and Zach are gaining."

"Why?"

"'Cause Rex is little, and Zach's... just gaining."

"Why do I get the feeling there's something you're not telling me?"

Brandon shrugged. "We're only thirteen or fourteen. We're supposed to be gaining weight. Like, it's totally normal."

"Gaining weight to grow is normal, but kids getting fat on

252

purpose is weird. I've seen those sites you bookmarked... 'gainers, feeders, encouragers.' Fat little kids showing off their bellies and playing with their boobs."

"The mook you been doing on my computer!"

"Mine crashed the other night," said Chad. "I'm calling the Geek Squad today. But I think you're evading the question. Why are *you* getting fat?"

Brandon looked down at himself. "Don't you like me this way?"

"So you admit you're getting fat?"

"Maybe a little. So?"

"You're still the same detestable brat, there's just more of you not to like. But girls won't think you're cool. And neither will most other people."

Brandon flexed an arm. "Check out these 'ceps. Paddling a long-board is hard." He puffed his chest. "Feel my pecs."

"Yeah, cute. You got some muscles under your chub. But, what good are muscles if no one can see them? It's like having money but dressing poor. ...How much do you weigh anyhow?"

"I dunno. The batteries are dead on our scale."

"Use mom and dad's, you might be surprised. ...And what did you do to your hair?"

"Just stopped parting it in the middle."

"But why is it getting all bushy and wild? Looks like an old-fashioned mop."

"Saltwater, I guess. ...I'm starting to get pretty good at surfing. And you should see Travis."

"That must make an interesting picture. Like, for Ripley's Believe It Or Not."

"Dork!"

Chad shrugged. "Surfing gives you a few cool points, but you have to start getting good at something that's going to make you money."

"Like learning to run the race?"

"He who dies with the most toys wins. ...So, what about your love life?"

"That's why I'm in the shower with you."

"It won't improve if you get fatter. ...So, what are you doing for Halloween?"

"Interesting segue."

"Halloween... trick-or-treat... candy... fat? But surely you're not going trick-or-treating... infantile as you still are?"

"Don't call me Shirley."

"That's so old it needs a walker."

"Tommy's taking Ro around here."

"No doubt the treats in this neighborhood blow off the low-budget crap in the Flats. But don't tell me you don't have plans to get mooked in some juvenile way."

"Like you don't?"

"Are you evading again? You know mom and dad will be gone overnight."

"So will you if you're smart," said Brandon. "Crash at somebody else's crib. The cops are setting up roadblocks to check for drunk drivers this year."

"I've just got muscles, I'm not retarded. ...And you?"

"I'm having a party with all 'those friends.'"

"What if I said no?"

"C'mon, Chad! It's just gonna be lots of food. Nobody's into drugs."

"Apparently not even diet drugs. But there'll be forties, of course?"

"And of course you'll take your commission."

"It's the American Way. Did you run it by mom and dad yet?"

"Maybe at dinner tonight. If they get home in time. ...And what was mom talking about just now when she said 'a year of public school?'"

"Oh dear, you weren't supposed to know that."

"You mookin' traitor!" yelled Brandon. "You knew all the time, didn't you?"

"No I didn't, swear to god. I just heard them talking the other night. They're trying for damage control."

"So I won't end up like you?"

"Don't push it, man, I might be on your side."

"...Why would you be on my side?"

"Because, oddly enough, I'm starting to like you... fat little clueless twink that you are. Don't talk about it unless I'm there. ...Back to the subject at hand: they'll say no alcohol, and they'll make you promise. You're not gonna walk on a technically like you did last time."

"I'll cross my fingers and lie like you."

"Wait till they have a few drinks. They might forget to mention it. Never lie if you can evade."

"So, it's cool with you, Chad?"

"Get down on your knees and beg... no don't it's far too Freudian. And remember what I said about how to handle drunk little kids."

"Rex is sleeping over."

"No doubt his jammies still have feet. ...*Assuming* I let you have this party, I'll call you until I get too mooked, but after that you're on your own." Chad glanced at his watch. "Okay, chubby, you've washed off your sins, now get your ass out of my shower."

TWENTY-EIGHT

Brandon dried himself with a designer towel, checked its label -- MADE IN HAITI -- then padded back to his room. His belly bobbed about as he walked and that felt kind of cool, like a part of himself he'd just discovered and could be enjoyed. It did seem bigger this morning, and its weight more noticeable.

He paused at the mirror to study himself: his pecs had lost some of their squareness, were rounder but more prominent suggesting softer boy-breast shapes. He remembered what Tommy had said: if he got fat he might look like Bosco. If Bosco had chosen to wear bigger shirts, update his style with an oversize look, he could have passed for a muscular dude... like getting the gain without any pain. Brandon's hair now resembled Bosco's, stiff with salt and porcupine spikes, but he hadn't changed it to copy Bosco; it was just simpler to wear it that way.

He dropped to the floor and did twenty push-ups; nothing soft about his muscles, though his belly bowed his back and bounced upon the carpet. But, more mass to lift would make his arms stronger. Travis probably looked like Kelvin under all his blubber. Brandon wondered if Travis would change if suddenly stripped of a few hundred pounds. Would he still write stories and read books?

There was nothing cool about being smart in the present place and time: the dumbing-down of American kids and waging a war on obesity by teleprompting them into zombies... lean, mean, unthinking things physically fit for work or war, who never questioned their masters' commands to buy and consume everything on the planet and hate anyone they were told to hate. Zombies ate brains of those who still had them, and being brainless was contagious.

256

He did more push-ups until he was sweating, then got up and switched on the stereo. He'd bought a Surfaris disk last week, happy teens singing of surf and sun, not about hating or killing each other. He opened the drapes on the patio door to greet a gray and foggy morning. It was hard to believe September was gone and Halloween only a week away.

He remembered what Chad had told him, about looking back from three years later upon the summer that changed everything. But you didn't know that till a long time after. Like seeing the ghost in that story, when you didn't *know* it was a ghost until a long time after. ...But *when* was it time to join the race? To get down with the fact that most of the things that mattered in life would happen somewhere between skateboards and wheelchairs; between beer-bongs and Ben-Gay for arthritis; between rock concerts and hearing-aids? Was it like the words in that Pink Floyd song: *No one told you when to run... you never heard the starting gun.*

So much in life required running -- at least in the metaphorical sense -- and whether you wanted to or not.

He heard the garage door rumble open, and his parents driving away to join the race over the hill. Then Chad's Trans-Am went squealing off to run the race at school.

He went to the window and parted the drapes: the sea was barely visible shrouded in silvery fog. A surfer rolled by on a skateboard, cutting school to go off the Point, choosing not to run the race.

"Pray for surf, dude," Brandon murmured.

He checked his emails: several more chubby boys wanted to cam, comparing their bellies and bodies with his and asking to see his face. That was the second stage of a friendship; first you showed off your body and talked to find out what you had in common besides just liking fat, then you trusted your friend with your face. It was cool to be getting compliments instead of being snubbed or ignored. No longer boringly Brandon. He'd made a lot of new friends on the web, and if he woke up in the dark lonely hours there was always some-body to talk to.

Kids in Australia were gaining, and in the U.K. and Germany. Also in Russia, Holland and France. There were lots of fat kids in Portugal,

Italy and Spain, and they didn't seem to be hated. He'd met several gainers in Argentina, Mexico, Bolivia, Saudi-Arabia, India, Canada and Greece. Also some in African countries, Vietnam and Denmark. And he'd heard more rumors, or urban legends, about immobile kids.

Someone pounded the patio door. Brandon went over, flipped the latch, and Troy staggered into the room. He was clad in nothing but gym shorts and sneaks, gasping for breath and pouring sweat. He stumbled and Brandon caught him.

"Hey," said Brandon. "What's the matter? You look like you're gonna croak."

"I'm cool," wheezed Troy. "Just lemmie... sit down... for a minute."

Brandon helped him to the bed. "Want some water?"

"Nah," panted Troy. "Water makes flab."

"No it doesn't, it just adds mass."

"But it looks like fat."

"Running again, wonder-boy?"

"...Yeah," puffed Troy. "Twice to the Bridges... and back... from the Point. ...After my... morning workout."

"Excuse a retarded question, but *why*?"

"*Only* a retard would ask that. ...Look at me, man."

"Yeah, you could star in a movie... I Was A Healthy Teenage Zombie... if you don't have a heart-attack first."

"Exercise is good for your heart."

"Then yours must be happy as mook," said Brandon, pressing a palm to Troy's jutting pecs. "Feels like a disco in there."

"That's 'cause it's getting stronger." Troy searched his shorts. "Get me a *little* glass of water."

"What are those?" asked Brandon, as Troy produced a small brown bottle.

"Fat burners."

Brandon frowned. "Those things are nothing but uppers, dork."

"No way!" panted Troy. "They're only sold to body-builders on the fitness web."

"And anyone else with a piece of plastic. How about some OJ? It would be better for you."

"Orange juice is fattening. It's one of the worst things you can drink if you're trying to watch your weight."

"So, excuse me for being retarded, but why should you have to watch your weight? Because you think everyone else is? That's kinda like paranoia."

"You saying it's sick to wanna be healthy?"

"I'm saying it's sick to *obsess* about health. To worry about how much you weigh all the time... like every pound more makes you less of a person. And what other people might think of your body."

"I don't want people to think I'm fat!" Troy studied Brandon. "Like you're getting. You need to start watching your own weight."

"I don't want to watch my weight," said Brandon. "There's too many other things to watch... like my back when I'm at school, so I don't get a beat-down, or shot or stabbed. Or get raped in P.E. by big healthy jocks with sick little minds. Not to mention lockdown drills in case of an average massacre. I have to watch bangers, crack-heads and bullies. I have to watch drug dealers, racists and haters. I have to watch teachers who shouldn't be teaching, and TV news that lies to me. I have to watch a government that tries to scare me with terrorist threats so it can make wars for oil. And greedy assholes who mook up my planet so they can die rich and leave me with shit. The *last* thing I'm going to watch is my weight and join the sick race to be 'healthy' so I can sweat and suffer like you to look like I'm told I should look."

Troy cocked his head. "You trying to write a book?"

"Maybe I am," said Brandon. "Call it The New Holy War... the war being waged for the new god of 'health,' a xenophobic, narcissistic god who encourages people to worship their bodies and hate anyone who doesn't... which sounds like something Satan would think of. And I'm doing my research by watching what I *should* be watching instead of what I'm told to watch. Like an 'obesity epidemic,' which is totally retarded. Like getting fat is some kind of disease you can catch from fat people... or another kind of terrorist threat. Like, forget what's *really* wrong with the world; you have to join the health-nazi party, become a lifestyle fascist... shoot me for

259

mixing metaphors... and fight the war on obesity. Like eating is some kind of dirty addiction and being fat means you're an addict. ...Like people who got hooked on drugs and spend their whole lives in 'recovery.' ...Like my uncle the alcoholic, who's scared to have a slice of rum cake or a brandy chocolate at Christmas because he might 'relapse.'"

Troy snorted. "You should know, stoner-boy."

"I stopped smoking dope because *I* wanted to, not because the TV told me."

Troy rolled his eyes. "Like you would say, wannabe writer, does this Ayn Randish rant have a point?"

"Life is too short to live in denial... denying yourself the good things in life by tying to prolong it instead of really living it; trying to stretch it another ten years with no guarantee you will. ...Like, food that tastes good is 'bad for your health' and might shorten the life you're trying to stretch. And the better it tastes the badder it is, so you should be scared of eating."

"You're really retarded, man," said Troy. "I'm not scared of eating."

"But eating is always resisting temptation instead of a normal thing you enjoy."

"Now what the mook are you talking about?"

"You always have to *think* about eating... like, what's 'safe' to eat and what's 'unhealthy.' And what you might like, but what you can't have... or what you've been told you shouldn't have. You're just like an addict scared of relapsing."

Troy snorted again. "My quality of life is better than yours because I'm living healthy."

"Is it?" said Brandon. "Check yourself, man, you're sweating gallons all over the place because you thought you had to run to preserve your quality of life... and don't bullshit me you enjoyed it. And you're scared of a glass of orange juice because you think it's a threat to the life you've been told is healthy. You've made eating perverted. Like a schizophrenic ritual; you have to do it a certain way or something bad will happen. And if you eat something you actually like, you have to feel guilty about it. It's not a normal part of your life."

Troy scowled. "And getting fat is 'normal?'"

"Getting skinny isn't. Not in nature, anyway. Losing weight means something's wrong... you're starving, sick, or dying. That's what your body thinks."

"Bodies don't think, brains think! And my brain controls my body." Troy poked Brandon's belly. "You're letting your body get out of control."

"Because I'm not starving it into submission? Or beating it into your kind of shape and shitting myself that's good for me?"

"It's like a little kid," said Troy. "You have make it obey, or it turns into a fat spoiled brat."

"You can also punish it too much and maybe it rebels."

"Oh yeah, like it's gonna run away. ...Just get me the water, okay."

Brandon went to the bathroom and got a glass of water. Troy swallowed three pills and washed them down. He'd almost recovered his breath by now, and wiped sweat from his face while scanning Brandon.

"You're really getting fat!"

"Oh, give it a funeral, Troy."

"Yeah, maybe yours! You better start taking care of yourself."

"You mean 'improving my quality of life' by denying myself what I like living for so I might survive another ten years and I can end up a healthy old corpse with the best-looking bod in the graveyard? The worms won't care how healthy I was, or all the good things I denied myself to prolong a life I *didn't* enjoy by doing what I wanted to do instead of what was 'healthy' for me by somebody else's standards. And I don't think God will either when He judges what kind of person I've been."

Troy shook his head, still breathing hard. "You'd think all that surfing would get you in shape."

Brandon flexed an arm. "Check that."

Troy squeezed Brandon's bicep and frowned. "Okay, not bad, but it doesn't show under all that flab."

"Which means I don't look healthy by your illustrated bible," said Brandon. "Which is what really matters to you, not how healthy I

261

actually am. But you'd better check the mirror, man, *you* look like a zombie with muscles. ...Not that I'm not glad to see you, but did you come here for some other reason except to sweat all over my bed and rag me about getting fat?"

"Can you check my English assignment? Like, for spelling and stuff?"

"Sure. Where is it?"

"You can read it on the bus."

"I've been taking Travis's bus. Or Bosco picks us up and we drop Ro at his school."

"Which is probably why you're getting fat."

"Maybe I'm also getting black."

"Zot?"

"If obesity is contagious, then being black must be, too."

"In Travis's case it could be both, and neither one is healthy."

Brandon sighed. "I know for a fact hate is contagious, and it's really an epidemic."

"How come you haven't come over lately?"

"You're always lifting weights. Or else you're running somewhere."

"You could run with me."

"How about skating like we used to?"

"Running is healthier."

Brandon sighed again. "Running to run is boring. If I take a walk or skate it's 'cause I want to go somewhere or have a little fun, not because it's 'healthy for me.' We're back to schizophrenic rites; fat is out to get you, so everything has to be done for 'health.'"

Troy shrugged. "Or maybe just an obtuse way of saying you found new friends this year."

"They could be your friends, too," said Brandon. "I'm having a party on Halloween and you know you're invited. ...Or, are you scared of pizza and beer? You ought to be in good enough shape to live a little once in a while. Like, what's the use of being healthy if you don't enjoy your life?"

"I got nothing in common with those dudes."

"You live on this planet, don't you?"

"I'm not saying Travis is stupid. And it's not his fault he's black."

"But, it is his fault he's fat?"

"Yeah it is," said Troy. "You told me about his genetic thing, but he could have his stomach stapled, or bypassed, or whatever it's called."

"I think I'd call it butchery, based on what I know. Or maybe a new kind of shock treatment, like they used to almost electrocute people to burn the craziness out of them. ...Hey, why not swallow a tape-worm? That seems about as medically advanced as cutting parts out of people to make them what they're 'supposed' to be."

"They cut out cancer because it kills you."

Brandon shrugged. "Maybe bypass is good for some people. Just about anything's good for somebody. But now it's becoming a style. There's a million doctors making billions redesigning people."

"Some people should be redesigned."

"By whose standards?"

"Obviously not yours, fat boy."

Brandon laughed. "I could have myself redesigned. Get my pecs squared-up like yours. Even get implants to make them bigger. Have my belly fat sucked out. Get all your gain without any pain. ...That's another reason to hate fat people; they can be happy being themselves, while you have to sweat and suffer and worry to be what you're told you should be."

Troy scowled. "Now what are you trying to say?"

"A lot of people are getting bypass because it's an easy way out of 'obesity.' ...As long as they can afford it. Isn't that the American Way? Get the work done without working yourself? ...And you make it sound like a final solution. Wanna make bypass mandatory for anyone you call obese? Which probably includes me now. ...And, wanna do lobotomies on anyone who doesn't agree? Who maybe... gasp!... likes being fat?"

"Nobody likes being fat!"

"Of course you know what 'everyone' likes, just like you know what everyone hates, and so did the real Nazis."

"If they do, it's sick and perverted!" snapped Troy.

"By the standards you've been *taught*. The ones you accept without asking why. And *that's* what's sick and perverted."

Troy shrugged. "Like I said, I got nothing in common with your new friends."

"How would you know if you never meet them?"

"I couldn't be seen with fat dudes."

"Not even Bosco?"

"I'm not into surfing anymore."

Brandon sighed. "You're invited to my party. Meet me at school in the library and I'll check your composition."

"Thanks." Troy got up but swayed on his feet and Brandon caught him again.

"Hey, Troy, you sure you're all right?"

Troy recovered. "Running just takes a lot out of me."

"So, try putting something back for a change. Let me get you that OJ, man. One little glass won't make you obese."

"Nah. ...But thanks. I gotta go shower."

"Slow down a little, dork. And eat some real food for breakfast instead of an 'energy bar.'" Brandon punched Troy's shoulder and smiled. "Even Arnold Schwarzenegger wasn't built in a day."

"He had some good ideas about health."

"Like concentration camps for fat kids? The government is watching your weight and telling you how can look? The master race *vill* be healthy... and will also dictate what 'healthy' is? Hitler said something like that... 'a german boy must be lean and mean, quick like a grey-hound and hard as Krupp steel.' And the Nazis took kids away from their parents if the kids weren't healthy by government standards... weren't fit to be good little Nazis. So, whatever happened to life, liberty, and the pursuit of happiness... individual happiness? ...Of course that didn't include slaves, or Native-Americans either, and now it doesn't include fat people."

Troy scowled. "You saying everyone should be fat?"

"I'm saying no one should be forced to be skinny, or be hated because they aren't."

"Since you put it that way, the master race should set an example."

"How about cleaning up the air the 'master race' polluted? And

264

saving the environment the 'master' race is killing? Or sharing food with starving people?"

Troy went to the door. "Obese people cost the government money."

"So do wars that never end. And caring for people made sick by pollution. Like all the kids with asthma today... which isn't caused by cigarette smoke."

"You think too much, Brandon."

"Maybe I do, which makes me a threat; so after they cut out part of my stomach, they'll cut out part of my brain."

TWENTY-NINE

randon's clean clothes, washed by the maid, were stacked on a chair by the door, jeans, boxers and shirts neatly folded, socks all properly paired. He remembered Bosco's messy room... he didn't have any drawers to fill; shorts in this one, shirts in that one, socks to the right and jeans in the bottom.

That was an interesting concept; when you had drawers and closets and shelves you had to have things to occupy them.

Maybe to justify your existence to people who judged you by things?

Brandon glanced around his room; every shelf crammed to capacity. Chad called the house a big empty barn, and yet it was totally stuffed with things, stuffed to obesity with things, even the rooms nobody used.

He snagged a pair of boxers and found them way too tight. That was okay, they were old. But even the newer ones pinched his hips. Shorts were kind of Capitalistic, another way to get your money for something you didn't really need. Bosco, he'd noted, didn't wear any.

He took his newest jeans off the chair. He'd bought them in August for school, and the knees and seams had faded a little, giving them just the right look. Then Tommy came in through the patio door dressed in jeans and a 'beater, the latter in typically Tommy style proudly showcasing his breasts. "Sup, Brandy-buck?"

"Did you see Troy going home?"

"Yeah. Is he sick?"

"Just high on health." Brandon pulled on his jeans. "So, how many pounds this week?"

266

"I'm not counting anymore." Tommy pulled up his shirt and bobbled his belly. "I'm free to be me and lovin' it." Then he sniffed the air. "Fee, fi, foe, fum, is that the smell of Brandon's...?"

"Gross!" said Brandon.

"It's totally normal."

"Lots of things are totally normal, but lots of people won't admit it. Now I have to change the sheets."

Tommy checked the bed. "What did you do, save it up for a week?"

"Stop being nasty. ...Beans!"

"Sorry," said Tommy.

"It's not you, these mookin' jeans shrank. And they were just starting to look cool."

"They'll stretch a little," said Tommy. "Mine are always tight after washing."

"Check it out," said Brandon. "I can't even get the top button buttoned."

Tommy came over. "Let me help. Suck in your belly."

"It is sucked in."

"I mean all the way."

"It is all the way."

Tommy struggled with the button. "Houston, we have a problem."

"Mookin' right!"

Tommy fondled Brandon's belly as if he was fluffing a pillow. "Guess I never noticed this month... had my own probs in the body department... but you're actually getting fat. A few more pounds and you'll have a cool hanger."

"But these were my coolest jeans," said Brandon.

"Some poor kid will be so stoked when he finds 'em at the Salvation Army."

"The mook I'm gonna give 'em away! ...I'll just stop eating lunch for a while."

"Or you could run with healthy-boy Troy."

"Ha, ha."

"Just leave a couple of buttons open and turn down the tops like

267

this." Tommy lifted his shirt and hoisted his blubber.

"I thought those jeans were new?" said Brandon.

"They are. But they don't make this style any bigger. You have to learn to adapt when you're fat."

"I *won't* have to learn to adapt, because I'm not getting any fatter."

Tommy looked thoughtful. "Remember that book, *Interview With The Vampire*? Like, on that first night when he was changing? Turning into something new? He was scared and confused."

"I'm not scared and confused. I just don't wanna buy new jeans; I need my money to roll our beast-feast."

"No prob, I can get us some money."

"...Doing fat vids?"

"Me and Ro got an act together and it's raking in green."

"I still think that's a little perverted."

"We don't do anything sexual."

"Isn't everything sexual according to Doctor Freud?"

"A cigar is whatever you want it to be."

"What do you do?"

"Feed each other Twinkies and cupcakes and get real messy doing it. Try to get into clothes that won't fit. Do the Truffle Shuffle and Milkshake... oldies but always goodies. Or, Ro pretends he's too fat to get up so I have to help him. You could join us if you wanna make money."

Brandon sighed. "Seems like I have to make money whether I want to or not."

"It's the price we pay for growing up... whether we want to or not."

"But I'm not *that* fat."

"Some people like to see skinny dudes interacting with fat ones. 'Specially feeding them or helping move all their fat around. It's a popular fantasy."

"Hey, I'm not skinny."

"Relatively speaking. ...Or, we tie you up in a chair and me and Ro stuff you with food. That's a good one, too, 'cause a lotta kids fantasize about somebody making them fat."

268

"But then I *would* get fat."

"Wouldn't that be good research? Then you'd know how it feels being fat... being inside instead of outside. And how you'd look... say if you got as fat as Bosco."

Leaving the top button open, Brandon sat down to put on his socks. "He isn't *that* fat."

Tommy smiled. "Isn't he a perfect fat kid like me?"

"I think I'd just call him the perfect kid in a Caucasian incarnation. Like, maybe a chubby Huck Finn."

"So, go with that," said Tommy. "I think you'd really look like him, too. 'Specially now with your hair all moppy."

Brandon glanced in the mirror, then studied Bosco's surfing picture.

"Admit it, Brandon, you're curious. You and Bosco are built the same, and you're both about as tall. Your faces even look alike. You just don't show your teeth as much."

"I don't smile as much as him."

"That's 'cause you're not as happy as him."

"He's happy *because* he's him. Because he's the star of his own movie, and because he likes his life, not because he's fat."

"Which is the best kind of happy to be."

Brandon shrugged. "Bosco's a champion surfer. He's good at something, and he's cool."

"You rock at writing and you're cool... 'least to people who appreciate you."

Brandon shrugged again. "Most people don't admire writers, they only admire a writer's work... assuming that work is any good. Most writers don't live exciting lives, and they're usually not exciting people. Or even cool sometimes."

"I thought great writers had to suffer?"

"Depends on what they write about. Like, if you're trying to make the world better, you should experience what's wrong. Mr. Akida suffered, and what he wrote helped things get better."

"But it didn't make him rich."

"You don't get rich by telling people they're ignorant haters and brainwashed fools." Brandon considered. "Even if I can be a writer, I probably won't be published for years. Not till I'm old, like twenty or something. I still have four years of high school ahead."

"So have a cool next four years."

"But I'm getting fat... at least a little."

"So, be a cool fat kid."

"That's an oxymoron these days."

"Only to actual morons."

"So, I should get fat so I can suffer? So I'll know what suffering is? Why don't I paint myself black instead?"

Tommy laughed. "I don't think you're ready to suffer *that* much."

THIRTY

"All right, Mr. DeMille, I'm ready for my close-up," said Brandon, coming into Tommy's room through its French patio doors, which overlooked a swimming pool half the size of his. He was clad as Tommy had prescribed in nothing but short cutoff jeans, a ragged old pair from his thirteenth summer that strained skin-tight on his thighs and bottom despite being only half-buttoned, enhancing the newly-gained roll of his belly lolling over in front.

Tommy's house was much older than Brandon's, one of the first on West Cliff Drive, in a stucco sort of Spanish style, and probably not quite worth two million despite its equal ocean view. Like most normal kids', Tommy's crib was a mess, a slightly smaller rendition of Brandon's with stereo, TV, computer and games, walls plastered with posters of classic rock bands – The Stones, Pink Floyd, Cream, and Led Zepplin – along with several of cute Ewoks, and big color copies of Travis and Ro. Also Bosco's magazine cover. It had been a couple of weeks since Brandon had last come over, and Tommy had added a Sony camcorder mounted on an aluminum tripod and looking film-maker professional. There were also two cone-shaded lights clamped to the dresser and bookshelf and aimed at Tommy's king-sized bed, which uncustomarily boasted a virginal-looking snowy-white sheet that made a dramatic contrast to Roosevelt's rolly midnight mass comfortably sprawled against big fluffy pillows. Ro was eating crème-filled cupcakes while watching *Ed, Edd and Eddy* on the fifty-inch TV, his boy-breasts like ebony melons of Jell-O bobbing about to his movements. At first Brandon thought he was naked because of the awesome bulk of his belly cascading over

271

mammoth thighs almost to his dimpled knees, but caught a glimpse of faded cutoffs under all that fat.

"Yo, Ro," said Brandon.

"Hey," said Ro, reaching for a gallon of milk on the beside table. "Want some cupcakes?"

"Don't we eat 'em when we're..." Brandon glanced at the cam, "performing?"

"We have tons of food," said Tommy, also in nothing but cutoffs – his old pair, Brandon noted, burst at the seams and baring plump thighs – and seated at his cluttered desk while scrolling his computer screen. "Hope you're hungry, we got ten requests; and mom's on a power-shopping spree so we have lots of time."

Ro gulped milk and wiped his mouth. "Better say we're booked-up for the rest of the day."

"Yeah," agreed Tommy, clattering keys, "or we'll pop for sure!"

"...Um?" said Brandon.

"Cigars," said Tommy.

Ro offered the milk jug to Brandon and laughed. "If I pop *that* way it don't show, so we're still E-rated, but I get a goofy look."

"...But, I thought you were only eleven?" said Brandon.

"Another fat secret," said Tommy. "Some fat kids puber early."

"Yeah, and it's bitchin'," said Ro.

Brandon took a swig of milk. "I thought this was just good clean fun."

Tommy shrugged. "Unless you have a dirty mind, in which case the whole world is dirty, like seeing life through smut-colored glasses."

Ro patted his undulant blubber. "Like I said, nobody can see it, so if I start lookin' goofy just keep doin' whatever you're doin' 'cause the show must go on."

"If we wanna get paid," added Tommy.

Brandon glanced at the camera again. "Some people would call this kiddie-porn."

Tommy rolled his eyes. "Some people call Harry Potter satanic."

"You do have a ton of food," said Brandon, passing the jug back to Ro and checking the mountain of snacks on the nightstand.

Besides many packs of cupcakes, there were Twinkies, Ding-Dongs, Gansitos and Ho-Hos. Also two aerosol cans of whipped cream and a big bottle of baby oil. "We're gonna eat all that?" he asked. "Though presumably not the oil."

"What we don't end up wearing," said Tommy. "Which does include the oil. We'll do the shower scene last for reasons which will become obvious."

"...Shower scene?" asked Brandon.

"Just good clean fun," said Ro, taking one of the whipped cream cans and jetting a Freudian spurt on his chest. "An' even if I pop, nobody can tell the difference on cam."

"...Could you warn me if you're gonna do that?"

Tommy laughed. "He won't, but watch for his goofy look."

"Excuse me for asking," said Brandon, as Ro wiped his breasts and licked his fingers. "I know you're mature for your age, and I don't mean just physically, but you *do* know what you're doing?"

"The whipped cream was my idea," said Ro. He jetted another spurt into his mouth so his cheeks puffed out like a chipmunk's, then swallowed and added, "An' Travis said it was cool."

"Oh," said Brandon. "So...?"

"We'll start simple," said Tommy. "Since you're new at this: A basic feed-the-fat-kid flick."

"That'll be me," said Ro. "An' make it hella messy."

"To make you get fatter?" asked Brandon. "Ostensibly, anyway."

Ro laughed. "Give the people what they want... 'least the ones who wanna pay."

Brandon leaned over Tommy's shoulder to scan a list of requests, and pointed. "Is *that* one from a kid?"

"Twelve," said Tommy. "And he's a regular customer."

"Skinny, I assume?"

Tommy pulled up a picture of a shirtless rusty-haired, freckle-faced boy who looked like a starving Opy Taylor serving time in the Mayberry jail... or maybe a Nazi death camp. "And his 'rents wanna keep him that way; calorie-count everything he eats, no spending-money to buy any snacks, and put him on a scale every day."

"Sounds like he's in a rehab program, or on parole for some-

273

thing."

"His 'rents are just proving they love him by not letting him get obese."

"So, watching us feed Ro is like fulfilling a fantasy of getting fat himself?"

"Basic post-pubescent rebellion against what his parents forbid him to do... which is often only perceived as being cruel and unusual, but in this case actually is."

"So he fantasizes about getting fat?"

"That's the most likely cause and effect; and a lot of gainers start in college when finally free of their parents' control. But he's also forbidden to have fat friends, so this might be just a way to have them." Tommy checked the screen again. "Funds transferred, lets give him good value; and he already knows the back-story."

"You have back-stories?" asked Brandon.

"Usual stuff... no pun intended: Ro's my BFF from next-door."

"Thought I was."

"Call it an alternate universe."

"So who am I in this one?"

"You can be Tommy's big brother," said Ro. "You come in and see him stuffin' me and wanna to do it, too."

"Like, it gets me excited?" asked Brandon.

Tommy laughed. "Didn't stuffing Zack do that?"

"There were other factors involved."

"Just remember this isn't for X-tube."

"Play with my fat a lot," said Ro. "Jiggle my boy-breasts and wobble my belly. The customers really like that."

"And watch for his goofy look," said Tommy.

"Are you gonna do that when you're stuffing me?"

"We'll watch for your goofy look," said Ro.

"...I don't get a goofy look."

"Yeah, you do," said Tommy, "like Scooby having a snack." He patted Brandon's belly. "We'll do the best we can with what little we have to work with."

"Hey!"

"Wait till me and Ro get started, then come in stage left and watch for a minute so the viewers identify."

"We won't know you're watchin'," said Ro.

"What are my lines?" asked Brandon.

"Just be yourself and improvise like you were writing a story," said Tommy. "Or, imagine you just came over not knowing what was going on."

"That will be fairly authentic," said Brandon.

Ro added, "Keep sayin' stuff like, you're so fat!"

Brandon smiled. "That's easy, you are."

"There you go."

"Then we'll overpower you," said Tommy.

"With all our fat," added Ro. "Then we tie you up in the chair an' start makin' you fat."

"Wouldn't that be fatter?"

"Most things are relative," said Tommy.

"Is this gonna be live?"

"No, we always edit," said Tommy. "In case something shows that isn't E-rated, but the audience thinks it's live." He got up and went to the cam. "We'll start on wide-shot automatic and do the close-ups later."

"An' use the Twinkies," said Ro. "They work better with my complexion."

"And remember we're all young mammals," said Tommy. "So don't get confused if you feel like a beast."

"Are you sure I'm not gonna need therapy?" said Brandon, going to the doorway.

"This is therapy," said Tommy. "Lights, camera... action!"

275

THIRTY-ONE

"Check it out, Brandon, they got Sumo suits."

Brandon looked where Tommy was pointing, seeing a mammothly fat mannequin with a chest like a pair of soccer balls and a gigantic blimp of a belly. It was naked except for a white loincloth and complete with a mop of black hair, though its color was blatantly racist, reminding Brandon of comic books published during World War II in which Japanese soldiers were cowardly yellow with Coke-bottle glasses and jutting rat-teeth.

"It's insulting to Asians," he said.

"Yeah," agreed Tommy, leading the way through the many people crowding the goth and costume shop. "They could have made it a normal color, but you can insult anybody who's fat."

As if to prove that, a wiry dude of maybe fifteen spun around as Tommy brushed by. "Watch who you're shovin', obese little pig!"

Brandon scowled. "Hey, man, he said excuse me. You deaf besides being an asshole?"

"If he wasn't so fuckin' obese he wouldn't need all the room!"

Brandon scoped the boy, noting adornments of obvious pride. "If you weren't such a fuckin' flamer you wouldn't be such a little bitch."

The dude checked Brandon, who was wearing an XL black T-shirt that made him look husky instead of chubby, maybe decided he couldn't take him, then muttered "hater!" and stalked away.

It was the day before Halloween and the store in Capitola Mall was swarming with all kinds of people from middle-school kids to middle-aged couples searching for costumes and alternate gear to show off their secret identities. Brandon didn't need anything

276

because of his party's Beastworld theme, but Travis and Ro had wanted fur vests. Since both were at work in their parents' rib shop, Brandon and Tom-my were shopping for them. They had checked the punk and gothic joints along Pacific Avenue, but had taken a bus to Capitola because nothing they'd found was big enough. They'd been searching a rack of fake furs -- tiger, leopard, zebra, giraffe -- and had found a double-X cheetah vest that looked large enough for Ro. But Travis needed two more X's, and nothing seemed to come in that size.

Brandon had muttered, "This ostensibly sucks," while sorting through the remaining furs.

Tommy had shrugged. "It's hard to find anything phat when you're fat, like fat people aren't supposed to look phat."

"Here's a maybe," Brandon had said. 'Looks like part of a were-wolf suit. There's no head and it's tagged half price."

"But it's not a vest," said Tommy, watching as Brandon tried on the top, which looked like a big furry overcoat.

"Cut off the sleeves and it is."

"Think it's big enough for Travis?"

"He'd have to wear it open," said Brandon. "It would never zip over his belly. Maybe we can find a model? Some dude around Travis's size, and ask him to try it on."

"Most kids that fat would be scared to come here."

"Yeah," agreed Brandon. "The vicious circle."

Though only technically chubby -- except to the health-nazi party -- Brandon now felt he was part of the fat world and had been on the lookout for hate. Despite being geared for the white middle-class -- the most fanatic of all fat haters -- there were a few fat kids at the mall. Most looked happy and confident, but of course there was safety in numbers; either you hung with other fat kids, or surrounded yourself with fat-friendly friends.

But, none of even the fattest kids were anywhere close to Travis's size. Just like on the internet, the really fat kids didn't show them-selves much; nobody wanted to be hated, or let their pictures get loose on the web where they could be used for anything from moronic memes to perverted porn.

277

In regard to the possible latter, and despite Tommy's assurance that he wouldn't be confused, Brandon hadn't been sure what to think about making the vids with Tommy and Ro, which -- after pauses to set up new scenes -- had climaxed in sort of a Beastworld vignette with all of them tumbled on Tommy's bed in a wildly writhing kaleidoscope of feeding, feasting, and fondling with enough whipped cream to have shocked even Freud. Ro had looked goofy several times, especially during the oiling session with Brandon doing most of the oiling, *masseur*-like massaging Tommy and Ro in ways that emphasized all their fat – getting whispered directions – with extra attention to bellies and breasts, until both boys were gleaming. Then there had been the squishing scenes, with Brandon usually the squishee, which, accord-ing to Tommy, fulfilled the vicarious fantasies of many thinner viewers; though there had also been a request for Tommy and Ro to wrestle each other with lots of mutual squishing. Last had come the shower scene – also widely in demand with much manipulation of glistening fat – and Brandon's share of the total take had been a hundred dollars. Still, he had hesitated a day before broaching the subject to Travis. Maybe it was stupid, but he felt as if he'd gone all the way with a good friend's sister and owed him at least a confession. But Travis had only laughed and said he might join the fun next time... which would probably fatten the profits by at least a hundred percent.

Now, here at the mall, Brandon had studied the wolf suit top, trying to picture Travis. "You try it on. You're one of the fattest dudes here."

Tommy had laughed. "I just look fatter around all these skinnies." Then he'd spotted the Sumo suit.

"Why do you want to see that?" asked Brandon.

"If the wolf thing fits him, it's gotta fit Travis."

A girl's voice spoke: "That would be kinda big for you."

Brandon turned to a cute chubby girl. She was totally goth in a tight black dress that emphasized her voluptuous curves. A studded belt encircled her waist, and her feet were clad in ass-kicking boots with bright and deadly steel toes. Curly hair flowed over her should-ers, framing a round and cheerful face with a small button nose and

278

full pouty lips under large and long-lashed ebony eyes. Oddly, it seemed to take a moment for Brandon to realize she was black; as black as all her gothic gear.

"Um..." he said, conscious of cool. "You work here?"

"Yeah," said the girl. "Overtime since it's Halloween, which is cool because I need the money." She glanced at the Sumo figure. "They used to come in kid sizes, too, but we couldn't get any this year."

Brandon smiled. "Maybe they don't want kids wearing them?"

"Yeah," said Tommy. "'Cause they might think they look phat being fat."

The girl's eyes seemed to be scanning Brandon, as if they could X-ray his oversize shirt. Then she smiled at Tommy, who was wearing a 'beater way too small displaying his belly and boy-breasts in mocking defiance of hater glares. "You could be right," she said.

"Hey, I like you," said Tommy.

Brandon smiled again, hoping he didn't look stupidly shy. "We don't wanna buy one." He held out the wolf suit top. "But, could we try this on him?"

The girl gave him a curious look but didn't seem to think he was weird.

"I have a big friend," Brandon added.

"He means fat," said Tommy.

"But I kinda forgot how fat he is."

"Oh," said the girl. "Sure, go ahead."

Brandon handed the fur to Tommy. "Um, what school do you go to?"

"Santa Cruz High."

"Um... you a Junior?"

"Just a fat Sophomore."

"Cool," said Brandon. Then, words came out before he could think. "Are you doing anything for lunch?" For a second he almost kicked himself: it sounded so mookin' clichéd! But, the girl looked disappointed, and Brandon was almost surprised.

"I can't today, we're too busy."

"That sucks," said Brandon. "But, you work here all the time?"

"Evenings and weekends. I'll have more time after Halloween."

Brandon caught himself before swallowing. "Um... so... would you wanna have lunch? I mean, when you can? ...Or maybe dinner?"

"Don't forget movies," said Tommy.

Brandon stepped on Tommy's toe. "My name's Brandon."

"I'm Darla," said the girl.

"Like from *The Little Rascals?*"

"Not many people would make the connection."

"Um, is that cool?"

"Sure," said Darla. "I like that show. So does my mom, obviously." She looked down at herself and added, "This isn't a Halloween cos-tume."

Brandon smiled. "That's really phat."

Darla smiled back. "Thank you."

"What do you think?" asked Tommy, who'd gotten the wolf top on the Sumo.

"...Oh," said Brandon. "It should fit Travis, unzipped like that."

"Your friend must be really fat," said Darla.

Brandon laughed easily now. "Yeah, both ways." He almost added Travis was black, but that didn't seem important.

"He'll make a wicked werewolf," said Darla. "But that's just part of a suit. It's the only triple XL we had, and the bottom got lost some-where, but I can find a head."

"He just wants a fur vest," said Brandon, "so we can cut off the sleeves. ...It's for a party. A fantasy theme."

"I like that stuff," said Darla. "If it's not too Pokémon."

"Nah, it's beasts. Mutant beasts."

"I love mutants," said Darla. "They're usually hated or misunder-stood."

"I've noticed that," said Brandon.

"I can take off the sleeves, no extra charge."

"Boss," said Brandon.

"I like retro stuff, too."

"Bitchin'," said Tommy.

Darla glanced at her death's-head watch. "It should be ready by two o'clock."

"Want me to pay for it now?" asked Brandon.

"That's okay. Any dude who would shop for a friend is gonna be true to his word." Darla looked thoughtful. "Was he scared to come here?"

"Nah. He's a Beastworld prince, panther genes."

"What genes do you have? I'd guess snow tiger."

"Hey, you're right. Would you be a leopard?"

"How did you guess?"

"Leopards are always cool like you."

"Thanks." Darla smiled at Tommy. "Of course you're lion?"

"Yeah, a phat one." Tommy nudged Brandon. "We can have lunch at the food court."

Brandon asked, "Can I get you something, Darla?"

"That would be phat. Cheeseburger, fries and a Coke."

"Miss?" asked a middle-aged woman, who somehow looked like she jogged every day... and didn't enjoy it. "Do you have any Barbie costumes?" Then she gave Tommy a frown. "You should lose weight, you're obese."

"I'm not obese, I'm fat," said Tommy. "And I have better manners than you."

"I think there's a Barbie suit left," said Darla. "In a very skinny size I'm sure would fit you perfectly."

"Never mind!" snapped the woman.

"C'mon," said Tommy. "I'm hungry."

"See you, Darla," said Brandon.

"Later, Brandon."

"She's more like a fox than a leopard," said Tommy, as he and Brandon left the shop. "A real foxy lady, like that Jimi Hendrix song."

"A phat foxy lady," Brandon improved. "I can't believe I talked to her and didn't make a mook of myself. ...Did I?"

"Nah, you were pretty phat."

THIRTY-TWO

"**D**arla liked what she saw," said Tommy. "But you shoulda worn a smaller shirt to show off more of it."

Brandon glanced around at the people, many of whom were glaring at Tommy as he and Brandon walked through the mall. "Then I could get hated, too."

"You aren't really fat till you get hated, and not really phat if you give a mook."

"Maybe I should go to Ross and buy a smaller shirt?"

"Be good research," said Tommy. "Why didn't you ask Darla to the party? Zach's bringing Nikki, and Kelvin's bringing a girl, too. You said Carlos is bringing someone, and I'm gonna ask a girl tonight; the phat little fox from my school."

"It seems kinda... sudden," said Brandon.

Tommy rolled his eyes. "*Life* is sudden, Brandon. A lot of things happen before you know it and then they're gone forever."

"I'm starting to notice that." Then Brandon sighed. "Guess I was too shy to ask her. The only reason I asked her to lunch is I didn't have time to get scared."

"Scared of what?"

"Looking uncool."

"Perhaps you mean fear of rejection?"

"Sometimes they're synonymous."

They passed a chubby little boy walking beside his mother. Another woman came up to the mother, a look of helpful concern on her face. "You should make him lose weight if you love him."

The mother looked stunned for a moment, but then ignored the other woman. The little boy looked confused.

Tommy muttered, "Now he thinks his mom doesn't love him. It's like those health food ads that say, 'for mothers who care what their children eat.' So if you don't buy their bogus beans, then you don't care about your kids... subliminal conditioning."

"People can really be assholes," said Brandon.

"'Specially when they've been brainwashed to be."

Then Brandon noticed a crowd ahead milling in front of a game store. People peered in through the doorway and windows, many with smirks or disgust on their faces. "Maybe somebody got busted trying to boost a game?"

"Da Beast's only interest is lunch," said Tommy.

Brandon paused to look into the shop, then grabbed Tommy's arm. "Bucky to Beast, do we *ever* have fat!"

"Zot?" said Tommy. Then his mouth dropped open. "Woah!"

He bulldozed his way through the people like a small Caterpillar wrapped in foam rubber, with Brandon close behind. Brandon felt *déjà vu* again, like when he'd first seen Travis at school. As he'd thought that first morning in History class, maybe Travis wasn't the world's fattest kid... but the dudes in the store could have been!

They were somewhere in their early teens, but just so impossibly, awesomely FAT it was hard to estimate their ages, though he saw they were obvious twins. One was aboard an electric scooter, a morph of chair and shopping cart on a tricycle chassis, the kind that were furnished by the mall so handicapped people could cruise. But the boy was so fat the little machine was almost buried under his blubber. If Brandon had brought his journal along he would have been frantically scribbling notes: *He avalanched out of a straining shirt that couldn't begin to contain all his fat.*

Both boys were dressed -- which was almost a joke -- in white T-shirts and faded jeans, but the clothes were cartoonishly small, the shirts stretched almost transparent, while their sleeves rode high on blubber-bulked arms more massive than even Tommy's thighs. Like Travis, their jeans bared most of their bottoms, which looked like pale planets colliding, while huge rolls of fat encircled their waists, and their bellies hung below their knees. Their navels looked like railroad tunnels, while their breasts were enormous wobbly spheres that seemed about to burst their shirts. Their faces were as round as moons under shaggy mops of light blond hair, and their complexions were peaches-and-cream so they looked like mammoth Hummel boys.

At first Brandon thought the boy on his feet was pushing his brother's scooter. But, no, the boy was just so fat he was using the machine for support to walk.

For a moment Brandon wondered if they were wearing costumes, like realistic Sumo suits designed in Hollywood. Was this some sort of public service in the war on childhood obesity...

DON'T TAKE IT LIGHTLY OR THIS WILL HAPPEN!

Or, maybe an infommerical to pimp the latest diet scam...

PAY US TO KEEP YOUR KIDS' MOUTHS SHUT UNLESS YOU WANT THEM TO LOOK LIKE THIS!

Brandon looked around, half expecting to see a film crew, but there were only stupid people gawking at a pair of fat boys.

Again he wondered if the dudes were in costume, maybe for Halloween? How could young teens have gotten *that* fat!

But the pair of impossibly fat boys didn't seem to be acting, and their "costumes" clearly weighed a ton... at least metaphorically. They were grimly ignoring the stares and glares and seemed to be here on a mission... here because they had to be, not because they were young teen boys who'd simply come to a mall. It seemed obvious now why their clothes were so small... these were *real* immobile kids who probably seldom, if ever, left home.

"Those dudes have balls," said Brandon.

"Big phat balls!" said Tommy.

Brandon scanned the faces around him: the kindest expression he saw was disgust. The worst could have made him go postal. "All they need is pitchforks and torches!"

"Don't forget sheets," said Tommy.

The gigantic twins had found their objective, one of the latest fantasy games. It was high on a rack, and the boy on his feet was straining up to reach it. Somehow he managed to stand on his toes and gain another inch. This bared even more of his blubbery body, getting more snickers and hate...

"Bet you a dollar he can't."

"Nah, he'll have a heart attack."

"Their parents should be shot!"

"Oink, oink!"

"Sooooo-weeee!"

"Lock 'em up an' starve the pigs!"

"There should be a law against that!"

A pizza-faced clerk of maybe sixteen could have helped the boy, but though he was a bit pudgy himself he also wore a smirk. Naturally, the enormous boy had to let go of his brother's scooter in his efforts to reach the game. But then his twin backed into him. Brandon watched in something like horror as the boy fell down in a slow-motion way, frame-by-frame like a buffering vid, collapsing onto to the floor in a floundering flubber of rolls. He didn't try to save himself by grabbing onto the game rack, obviously knowing he'd just bring it down. Brandon heard him say, "oh, shit!" as several people laughed.

Brandon hurried over with Tommy, shoving their way through the slavering trolls.

"Hey, dudes," said Tommy. "What's up?"

The boy on the scooter looked wary, but then his expression changed to a grin. "Hey, you're Bucky an' Beast!"

"To da rescue," said Tommy, bowing.

"I need it," puffed boy on the floor.

"You okay?" asked Brandon, kneeling beside the mammoth dude.

"Yeah," said the boy. "But I'm too fat to get up by myself when there's nothin' to grab."

"Shut up, dork!" hissed his brother, looking around at the muttering mob. "Want 'em to call the fire department? Or maybe the freakin' cops?"

"Shit no!"

"Can you grab the scooter?" asked Brandon.

"Maybe," puffed the boy on the floor. "But it's gonna be funny to watch."

The acne-afflicted clerk had come over, looking more annoyed than concerned. "You all right?" he asked. (Fatso -- or probably worse -- seemed implied.)

"He's cool," said the dude on the scooter. "He was just trying to get that game."

"You could have helped," said Brandon.

Pizza-face scowled. "You givin' me shit? I'll call Security."

"All we want is the game," panted the boy on the floor.

"Go ring it up," said Brandon, snagging the game off the rack.

Tommy added, "And you better watch your store; something might get boosted while all these assholes are hating on us."

"...Yeah," said the dude, looking slightly more human. He turned to the boy on the floor again. "Sure you're okay?"

"Yeah. We just want the game."

"Cash or card?"

The boy on the scooter dug in a pocket and handed the clerk a Visa.

"Can we help you get up?" asked Brandon after the clerk walked away.

"If you don't mind getting' hated."

"Never been a prob for me."

"I can't help," said the boy on the scooter. "If I get down on my knees, you'll have to help *me* up."

"Yeah, big help!" puffed his brother. "You can't even drive that thing!"

"Bite me, dork! The reverse button stuck! Now, c'mon, get up. Or, do you *wanna* be on TV?"

Brandon shoved a shoulder under one of the boy's enormous arms. "Tommy, take his other arm."

"On it, Bucky."

It took several minutes of struggle to get the huge boy on his feet. At least twenty people were watching -- muscular teens, "healthy" adults -- but no one offered to help. At last the boy was vertical, or as much as he could be leaning way back to balance his belly, grasping the back of his brother's scooter, panting for breath and pouring sweat.

"Thanks, dudes," he puffed, and offered a hand. "I'm Ronny."

"I'm Donny," said the boy on the scooter.

"Tommy," said Tommy. "And this is Brandon. You dudes are mad, crazy bitchin' boss phat!"

"Don't start admiring now," said Brandon, eyeing the hostile crowd. "Sure as mook isn't the time and place."

"You admirers?" asked Ronny.

"Yeah, of cool people," said Brandon.

A woman snapped, "There should be a law against getting obese!"

A man growled, "You should have your stomachs cut out!"

A woman snarled, "Your parents should be put in jail!"

Brandon felt a flash of rage, and was glad he didn't have a gun, but then the clerk returned.

"You guys better leave." He handed Donny the game in a bag. "...Thanks."

"You're welcome," said Ronny.

Then, to his credit, the clerk faced the crowd. "Anybody who's not here for games, get out or I'll call Security!"

Most of the mob began to leave, muttering, snickering, shaking their heads. But a chubby boy of maybe ten flashed the twins a thumbs-up sign as Ronny waddled ponderously behind his brother's scooter.

"It's my turn now," panted Ronny when they were out in the corridor.

"You dudes should have two," said Tommy.

"The guard didn't wanna let us use 'em."

"Yeah," said Donny. "He said we didn't have to be fat so we didn't have any right to use 'em. We boosted this one when he went away."

Brandon scoped the corridor, seeing the glares, hearing the hate. "It really took courage to come here."

"Tons," said Tommy. "You dudes with your 'rents?"

"Nah," said Ronny, easing his bulk onto the scooter, its little tires

287

flattening under his weight.

"There's just mom," said Donny. "She works in Silicon Valley."

Ronny added, "She wouldn't believe we'd go out."

"Dad used to try an' make us," said Donny. "Like it says on TV, 'go out an' play for an hour every day.'"

"But, then he got divorced," said Ronny. "He hated us for being fat."

"Yeah," said Donny. "An' after we got over three-hundred pounds it wasn't safe goin' out anymore."

"We home-school online," said Ronny.

"How old are you?" asked Tommy.

"Thirteen," said Donny.

"I'm older," said Ronny.

Donny snorted. "By three minutes!"

"We can guess your next question," said Ronny.

"But we don't know," said Donny. "We weighed about four-fifty last year."

"Close to five," said Tommy, giving the twins an expert scoping. He added to Brandon, "They just look fatter than Travis because they're not as tall."

Brandon glanced at the game in the bag. "You must have hella wanted that."

"It just came out," said Ronny.

Donny added, "We mostly buy stuff on the web, but we wanted this one today."

"How did you get here?" asked Tommy.

"Bus," said Donny.

"That must have been an adventure," said Brandon.

Ronny nodded. "We forgot how many haters there were."

"We live in Santa Cruz Gardens," said Donny. "Wanna come over sometime? We got tons of games an' a fifty-inch screen."

"Def!" said Tommy. "Me and Brandon were gonna have lunch. You dudes wanna join us?"

The twins looked around at the people, who slowed as they passed to stare and glare.

"You made it this far," Tommy added. "The food court's just

288

around the corner."

"Well," said Ronny. "We can't get hated any more than what already happened."

"Unless you fall down again," said Donny.

"You backed into me, dork!"

Tommy laughed. "C'mon, all this hate is making me hungry."

With Ronny now driving the scooter and Donny waddling slowly behind, they started for the food court. A little boy of maybe six broke away from his mother's hand and began to follow them. "Fatty, fatty two-by-four couldn't get through the bathroom door!"

"That's original," said Tommy.

Brandon glared at the mother, who was doing less than nothing. "Would you let him yell nigger, beaner, or queer?"

The woman glared back. "There should be a law against getting obese!"

"There should be a law against parents like you who teach their kids to hate!" Then Brandon got in the little boy's face. "Skinny, skinny hater rat you're a stupid little brat!"

The kid looked shocked. "Mommy!"

Tommy laughed. "Bucky strikes back."

The twins laughed, too, but then Donny said, "Don't do that, she might report us."

"For what?" asked Brandon. "We should report her!"

Ronny shrugged. "It's safer not to fight back 'cause nobody's on your side when you're fat."

Brandon glanced at Tommy. "We are."

A few minutes later they reached the food court. "I'm buying," said Tommy. "What does everybody want?"

"Double cheeseburger," said Donny. He chose a corner table with a sturdy bench instead of chairs. "Fries, an' a root beer float."

"Clone it," said Ronny, driving the scooter up to the table.

"What about dessert?" asked Tommy. "Don't be shy, I can afford it."

"Um," said Brandon, glancing around at the scowling people. "That might be like throwing gas on a fire."

Donny laughed. "They'd hate us if we ate carrot sticks."

"We don't really eat much junk," added Ronny. "Mom makes pretty good stuff at home."

"You rich, Tommy?" asked Donny.

"We do fat vids," said Tommy, flicking a grin a Brandon.

"That pays good," said Ronny. "We just started doin' 'em."

Donny added, "It's how we made enough for the game."

Tommy laughed. "You dudes are so mookin' awesome you'll make enough to buy your own scooters."

"Then we better stay in shape. I'll have a banana spilt," said Donny.

"Clone it," said Ronny.

"I'll have the same," said Brandon. "Since Da Beast is livin' so large."

"I'll pay for Darla's, too," said Tommy and headed for the burger booth.

"Um?" asked Brandon, snagging a chair from another table. "Do you think you would have gotten so fat if people didn't hate on you? Like, made going out a torture? ...Ever feel like prisoners of weight?"

Ronny said, "We used to ride our bikes all over. An' go up in the hills."

Donny nodded. "An' down to the beach. We skated until we were almost eleven."

"Till the hate cranked up," said Ronny.

"Assholes yellin' from cars," said Donny.

Ronny nodded. "An' people tellin' us to lose weight everywhere we went."

"Yeah," said Donny. "Not "hey' or 'hi,' or what's your name, just 'go on a diet, pigs!'"

"Would you still do those things?" asked Brandon. "Go to the beach and stuff like that if people didn't hate on you?"

"Sure," said Ronny. "We miss the beach. An' we haven't been to the Boardwalk in years. We heard they updated the Cave Train."

"Same with goin' to movies," said Donny. "Like, *we're* the show, not what's on the screen."

Brandon was making mental notes. "So, it's not being fat that's stopping you from going out and doing stuff, it's all the stupid hate."

"You writing a book?" asked Ronny.

"Would you laugh if I said I was?"

"You're not laughing at us," said Donny.

Ronny looked around again at all the stares and glares; and the O-word seemed to echo like a chant in a church or a holy-war cry. "We're not prisoners of weight, just prisoners of hate."

Tommy returned with a heaping tray. "This is for Darla," he said, handing Brandon a paper bag.

"'Scuse me," said Brandon, getting up. "Back in a minute."

"Where you goin'?" asked Tommy.

"To ask a girl to a party."

"Aren't you still scared?"

"What do I have to be scared of?"

THIRTY-THREE

"**B**oss party, Brandon!" said Rex.

Brandon smiled. "*Déjà vu*."

"Oh yeah," said Rex, and gulped from his forty, his tummy a tumescent hemisphere protruding way over his sagging shorts and enhancing the childish sway of his back from being steadily stuffed since September. "But it sheems... seems, like a long time ago."

"Maybe it was," said Brandon.

They were standing in the kitchen doorway surveying the scene by the flood-lit pool. Indian Summer still ruled Santa Cruz, and the salt-scented night was sensually warm. Except for Tommy and Ro, who were still out Trick-Or-Treating, everyone else had arrived around seven, including Bosco with a case of Bud to back up Brandon's forties. Brandon had brought his TV outside and set it on a patio table. He'd rented some old-time horror movies, and *I Was A Teenage Werewolf* was playing. A feast of pizzas, chips and dips was spread on another table, along with platters of juicy ribs from Travis's parents' cafe. Travis wore the furry vest and looked like a mighty mutant prince. Danny was clad in a similar style, and Kelvin, Carlos, Nikki and Zach also wore fur and mutant gear.

Ronny and Donny had just arrived, rolling up in a minivan so overloaded by their weight its tail had dragged pulling into the driveway. The twins had looked surprised at the mall when Brandon had invited them... no one had asked them anywhere since they'd gotten over 300 pounds. But they'd waited to come until well after dark... America the Beautiful was having an ugly epidemic of hating people because of their size.

292

Their mother was a slender woman who could have been in the movies and hardly even looked old enough to have a pair of teenage sons.

Rex was dressed as Sonic, Kelvin as a Panther (of course), but Bosco wore only a sheepskin vest -- probably made from an ancient coat -- above his ragged cutoffs, which made him look like a shepherd boy among a flock of furries.

Brandon turned to smile at Darla, who was dressed as a gothic leopard girl and making a bowl of creamy ranch dip. "Hey," he said, "you don't have to do that."

Darla laughed. "I have three brothers, big fat brothers, so I'm used to feeding people."

Tommy came in from the hallway escorting his date, a cute chubby girl, and Ro came wobbling and quaking behind. All were dressed as mutant beasts and toted bulging bags of candy.

"Hey, Brandon," said Tommy. "This is Terri. Terri, this is Brandon."

"Hi, Terri," said Brandon.

Terri, Ro and Rex went out to join the other beasts, and Tommy grinned at Brandon. "Terri's a phat little fox, huh?"

"Even phatter dressed like one."

"Yeah, and check out her tail."

"Don't be crude."

"Sometimes a tail is just a tail." Tommy scanned the patio. "Ronny and Donny came. Cool!"

"Their mom seemed as surprised as they were that anybody would ask them," said Brandon.

"Did she apologize for their fat?"

"No, and she seemed... well, normal, and I don't mean her size."

"So are Ronny and Donny."

Brandon smiled. "I've noticed."

"Guess Troy didn't come?"

"I didn't think he would, but I was kinda hoping. I feel like I deserted him."

"I'd call it the other way 'round," said Tommy. "But sometimes that's part of growing up... people going different ways, like you said about time splitting."

"I think he's going the wrong way."

"And he thinks the same about you. ...Guess Jason didn't come either?"

"No, and that's kinda sad."

Tommy shrugged. "You reached out to him, and that's all you can do. Somebody has to want to be helped before anybody can help them. But I think Troy might have wanted to come."

"Why?" asked Brandon.

"When we were coming up to the house I thought I seen somebody."

"Saw somebody."

"Discerned somebody. Peeping through the fence in back."

"Think it was Troy?" asked Brandon. "Maybe checking what he was missing?"

Tommy shrugged again. "It was dark. I'm not even sure I saw anything; coulda just been a shadow."

"If somebody was, I hope it was Troy. I almost feel like we could get busted."

"For what?" asked Tommy. "'Using alcohol?'"

"Being fat and having fun. Like, we might get arrested by Homeland Health."

Darla finished mixing the dip. "Or lynched by the calorie KKK."

It was a peaceful party. Although there was plenty of beer and malt nobody got more than mildly mooked, though Rex fell asleep with a rib in his hand, and Brandon laid him to rest in the guest room... and not on his back. The twins had longingly gazed at the pool -- they hadn't gone swimming in years -- and had finally asked if they could go in. Brandon had thought about swimming, but this party *was* "mixed company," and somebody might have been spying on them... he'd gone out to check the backyard fence from the next-door neighbor's side and found some flowers trampled near a big knothole. It *might* have been someone spying, or could have just been some-body's dog sniffing out a gopher.

He wished he'd suggested swimming attire as alternate dress for his guests. The other dudes were in cutoffs or shorts, but Donny and

Ronny had only their jeans. The twins weren't shy -- they wore nothing at home -- but Brandon imagined the headlines:

CHILDHOOD OBESITY LINKED TO IMMORAL BEHAVIOR!
OBESE TEEN ORGY ON WEST CLIFF DRIVE!

Why not? Being fat was supposedly linked to as many bad things as being black.

But, Darla had reminded him of the dryer in the laundry room, which was something he never thought about since he didn't do laundry. There were plenty of towels in the house, so all the beasts went swimming in appropriate parts of their attire, then wore the towels while their clothes were drying.

Midnight came before Brandon knew it; and Danny's father had picked him up in a rusty 1970s truck. Zach's mom had come for him and Nikki; Carlos and his chubby date had caught a bus on the corner; and Terri's mom had rescued her from Tommy's beastly embrace. Travis's father had rolled up in a newly-purchased delivery van with Righteous Ribs on its sides. Travis had done the graphic, a fat black boy in cartoon style who was aiming a rib instead of a gun... definitely food for thought.

Tommy now sprawled in a patio chair, while Bosco sat on the edge of the pool with his feet in the glimmering water, the pungent smoke of his cigar ghosting about in the salt-scented air. Ronny and Donny, back in their jeans, were watching *Screaming Skull*, and Brandon and Darla were sitting together on a bench at one of the tables. Darla had asked about Brandon's writing... she wrote gothic tales. Probably with the aid of malt, Brandon had finally worked up the courage to take Darla's hand as they talked. He was thinking ahead to a possible kiss when the doorbell rang.

Brandon pressed Darla's hand -- implying (he hoped) his hope of a kiss -- then went to answer the door. He checked the monitor to be safe, but it was Ronny and Donny's mom.

"Come in," he said, opening the door. "They're out by the pool, we all went swimming."

The woman smiled. "I'm sure they liked that; and it was very nice of you to invite them tonight."

"I'm glad they came," said Brandon. "I'll go get them." He started across the living room, but the woman asked:

"Do you think I'm a bad parent?"

"Huh?" said Brandon, turning around. "Why would I think that?"

"I'd think it would be obvious."

"'Cause they're fat?"

"You didn't say obese."

"I don't use hate words except against haters."

The woman sighed. "They were chubby toddlers, but I never seemed to notice how fat they were getting as kids."

"You were seeing them every day," said Brandon. "Seeing *them*, the kids you loved, not how much they weighed."

"My husband saw their weight. Toward the... end... it was all he saw. And everything they couldn't do because they were 'obese.' But nothing they were good at doing... getting good grades, reading books, being happy intelligent kids... none of that mattered to him."

"It happens a lot," said Brandon. "Like, parents are basically saying I won't love you unless you lose weight. Like, there's a price for love by the pound, and the more you weigh the less you'll get."

"Some people would call that tough love."

Brandon shook his head. "There's no such color as 'light black;' it's either black or it's something else. And it's either love or it's some-thing else, and kids need the real thing."

The woman smiled. "You seem to have a way with words."

"I've thought a lot about being fat... lately anyhow. And the way it changes people's lives because *other* people obsess about it."

The woman nodded. "I've also been thinking about it a lot. Does it mean I don't really love my sons because I let them get fat? Which makes other people hate them."

"Only bad people hate," said Brandon. "Sick little people who *choose* to hate. ...You don't talk about stuff like this much. Huh?"

"There's no one to talk about it with. Not objectively. Of course there are thousands of weight-loss groups, support for parents with kids on diets, or kids about to have bypass, but no one seems to want to accept..."

Brandon smiled. "That some kids are fat and it's okay?"

"And there's so much pressure on their parents."

"To redesign their kids," said Brandon. "Like, you *vill* have skinny kids and if you don't we'll punish you."

The woman nodded again. "That's mostly what it's about. Nobody wants to defend fat kids, as if they have no right to be happy. No one cares if they're taunted and bullied, humiliated and ridiculed; and the same applies to their parents."

"Yeah," said Brandon. "Like, 'if you loved them you'd make them lose weight.' So, if they're fat it means you don't love them. And since you don't love them, you're a bad parent. It's the same kind of logic they use in commercials... 'our cereal is healthy for kids, so if you don't buy it, you don't love them.' It works with religions and governments, too... but only on people who've been taught not to think."

"You seem to know the story."

"I'm kinda doing research." Brandon patted his belly. "And maybe from the inside."

"My name is Lynda Carter. My mother loved *Wonder Woman*. ...That show from the 1970s."

"I've seen a few on the classic channel."

"I feel like I have to be Wonder Woman. When Ronny and Donny were born, I tried to prepare myself to protect them. First from all the baby dangers, with child-proof caps and car seats, safety plugs in electric outlets, a lock on the cleaning cabinet door. Then later from drugs and violence by teaching them to say no. And by teaching them to be kind and not to hate anyone. I was concerned about public schools. I wanted the best education for them."

Lynda smiled a little. "It's ironic that being fat is giving them better education. They'll graduate high school on-line next year, then they're starting college courses. They're already designing games, and a com-pany is interested. And it keeps them away from drugs and violence."

Then she sighed. "But not the hate. That seeps in on TV every day and leaks in from the Web. It's something that can't be parent-blocked no matter how hard you try."

"I know," said Brandon. "It's in everything from cartoons to commercials. Like, open season on fat kids and nobody needs a hater license."

Lynda sighed again. "Maybe I should have done something, made them feel bad about being fat like everybody says I should, threatened to send them to a fat camp, put them on diets or weight-loss drugs, said no to what all their friends were eating... McDonalds, pizza, cereals, snacks... all the things they see on TV."

"And are taught to want," said Brandon. "Making people want lots of food, and making them want to stay skinny, too, makes billions of dollars for industries. One side makes you get fat... or makes it easy for you to get fat... and the other side makes you want to get skinny. It's like a never-ending war of gain, lose, and control your weight that doesn't accomplish anything or make the world any better. It only wastes our resources by making people buy and consume over and over again like a loop. ...Like, eat a big dinner and then 'work it off.' That only means you've wasted the food... it's politically-correct bulimia... so why should people feel good about it? Or better than someone who didn't waste food because they let it go to their waist?"

"I've thought of that myself," said Lynda. "It's not promoting health, it's only pimping it like a product and exploiting the people who buy it. We accuse tobacco companies of preying on kids for future smokers, but the health industry does the same thing by making kids obsess about weight. ...And it is like a loop: a fast-food ad then a diet commercial, over and over again."

She glanced down the hall where Ronny and Donny were waddling in. "I cook healthy meals and give them vitamins. I've studied medicine and nursing. It's hard to find a doctor who doesn't make them feel bad. I thought 'do no harm' was a doctor's code, but hurting kids' feelings *is* doing harm. They can't find anything wrong with my sons except to say they're 'obese.' They prescribe pills or advise surgery. They tell me to put them on diets or send them away to weight-loss camps. ...Or even threaten to take them away. It's always as if they have a disease that has to be cured, controlled, or cut out."

"Yeah," said Brandon. "And they never admit what's *really* wrong is that most fat kids would be healthy if they could just go out and do stuff without getting hated and dissed all the time. Even good people don't understand they're only encouraging ignorant hate and helping both sides keep the war going on... and making money... by saying all kids should be skinny."

Lynda smiled. "You must be writing a book, and if you're not you should be."

"It probably wouldn't sell," said Brandon. "People don't like being told they're ignorant haters and brainwashed fools. ...I have a fat friend who goes to a doctor who's more concerned about how he feels than how much he weighs. I could hook you up with him."

"Thank you," said Lynda. "That's the kind of support I need." She hesitated, then asked, "Maybe it proves I am a bad parent, but do you think my sons are too fat?"

Brandon glanced at the huge boys lumbering up the hall. "A lot of people would say yes... they're too fat and you're a bad parent. But I don't know much about them... or you. I'd be like a million other fools who only judge them by their weight; who want them look how *they* think they should look. Or how they've been told to think they should look. I've only known them a few hours, but they seem happy to me. I don't think a lot of people are happy, no matter how healthy they think they are. It's easy to put the blame on you, and I guess a lot of people would. But those are the same kind of ignorant trolls who make it so hard for them to be happy, who won't accept they're just normal kids who happen to be fat... who won't let them be normal kids."

Brandon considered. "In their case that might have been an advantage, but for most fat kids it's a handicap that other people inflict on them... sometimes with the best intentions but usually with the worst."

Lynda smiled again. "It doesn't sound as if you're very normal."

"That's probably 'cause of my parents. Once upon a time they weren't normal, either."

"Once upon a time?"

Brandon glanced at a framed photograph of his mom and dad in their early twenties kissing on a beach. "They used to be kind of radical. Like freedom fighters, maybe. For human rights and things like that... life, liberty, and the pursuit of happiness. They were against discrimination based on color, religion or race. ...Guess they never thought about size. But maybe someday they'll start fighting again."

"I'm sure they will," said Lynda. "And maybe because of you. Thank you for listening to me. ...Would you happen to be looking for a part-time job a few hours a day after school?"

"I never thought about it," said Brandon. "'Cause I never had to. ...You mean with Ronny and Donny?"

"Yes," said Lynda. "They're alone so much with me working. They could get more exercise if they had somebody to do things with. There are miles of woods behind our house; they used to go exploring but now they're afraid to go out because someone might attack them, verbally or physically. It's been just about impossible to find anyone to be with them. The few people who can accept their size are usually older women who aren't very active themselves. And there's always a risk someone will report them. I almost had a heart attack when they told me they'd gone to the mall yesterday. And God only knows what might have happened if you and your friend hadn't been there."

Brandon smiled. "We're Bucky and Beast, we fight evil and hate. And so do the other mutants I know. ...And, yeah, that would be a cool job. And they could come here and swim in the pool." He turned around as the twins arrived. "Have a good time?"

"Bitchin'!" said Donny.

"Boss!" said Ronny.

They waddled out to the minivan and loaded themselves in the back. Brandon, Darla, Tommy and Bosco waved goodbye as the van rolled away. The lighthouse flashed its beam on the Point; the neighborhood lawns glistened with dew; and a sea lion barked in the distance.

"Guess I should be going," said Darla. "Your party rocked, Brandon."

"Thanks, but you helped rock it." Brandon offered his hand. "I'll walk you to the bus stop. ...Um, can I see you tomorrow? Maybe have lunch at the mall?"

"I'd like that," said Darla. Then she leaned close and kissed Brandon's lips, sending a tingle of warmth through his body.

Brandon had hoped for a little more, but that was enough... at least for this time.

THIRTY-FOUR

Tommy was yawning when Brandon returned. "See you for breakfast, Bucky."

"'Night, Beast, sweet dreams about Terri."

"Wet ones I hope!" Tommy laughed as he headed for his house.

Brandon turned to Bosco, beside him and gazing out at the sea. "Guess you don't have a curfew?"

"Time don't mean nothin' when you're havin' fun."

Brandon smiled. "I think I'm starting to notice that, and I think there's a couple beers left."

Bosco grinned his beaver grin. "Always time for beer."

"Wanna sit by the pool?" asked Brandon. "I should check on Rex."

"Sure, Brandy-buck, I'll get the brew."

Brandon peeped into the guest room, where Rex was sleeping peacefully, then went out on the patio. Bosco sat on the edge of the pool, his feet in the water, a bottle in hand, another waiting for Brandon. He offered cigars as Brandon sat down, and fired them with a wooden match. They smoked in silence, sipping beer, as crickets chirped in the flowerbeds and the sea murmured softly against the cliffs.

Brandon saw his and Bosco's reflections mirrored in the quiet pool. For a moment he thought there were two of himself. He recalled what he'd felt at the last party when Bosco had rolled up the drive-way on a wooden plank with steel wheels and he'd pictured a long-vanished time. Or maybe a future that should have happened. ...And maybe, just for a second, had he actually gotten *there*? He studied the boys in the water; his hair wasn't quite as bushy and

302

wild, his face not as round, his chest not as chubby, his belly concealing less of his lap. Then he faced the boy beside him, like looking into an alternate mirror where things were the same, but not quite the same. He touched Bosco's arm. "Who are you, man?"

Bosco smiled his careless smile. "Just me, myself an' I, same as always."

"But weren't you ever confused?" asked Brandon. "Like, didn't know who you really were... or maybe who you thought you should be?"

Bosco puffed out a ghost of smoke. "Never thought about who I should be 'cause I like bein' who I am, even if that ain't all I could be, but maybe I just ain't finished yet." He threw an arm over Brandon's shoulders like boys used to do in *Leave It To Beaver* before they'd been taught it might mean something else. "An' I meet good people who like me for me, so why would I wanna be anyone else?"

Brandon felt attraction again, like what Tommy had talked about, and what he'd felt in Bosco's room seeing him asleep. He suddenly felt like the evil Beastmaster, alone in his lab with a young mutant boy who'd just woken up and was innocent.

"Um," he said, with a husky reluctance before he asked what he wanted to ask, "guess it's getting late, man."

"Or maybe early," said Bosco. "Sometimes you can't the difference."

Brandon got to his feet with the other boy and walked with him out to the van, feeling a longing for something he'd lost as Bosco got in and drove away.

Or maybe for something he might never find?

303

THIRTY-FIVE

Brandon was in that timeless place out beyond the breakers. He was sitting astride his gift from Bosco, the ancient longboard with its fierce tiki god. The sky was clear and blue above, and the water was liquid emerald. He gazed into the crystal depths and saw his mirror image. He seemed to be rising to meet himself, then realized it was Bosco. He offered a hand to help Bosco aboard, glistening brown in the golden sun like a rolly-poly sea-lion pup.

"Dude, we're there," said Bosco, facing Brandon astride the board.

Brandon embraced the other boy, feeling his arms go around himself, feeling his chest against his chest in a time and place he'd always been.

"Brandon!"

Brandon opened his eyes. Morning sun glowed on the window curtains, softly lighting his room. Then he heard a siren, maybe down at Lighthouse Point but rapidly approaching. Chad stood at his beside still dressed as he'd been when he'd left yesterday.

"What's up?" asked Brandon sleepily.

"What happened last night?" Chad demanded.

"...Huh?"

"At your party! ...Wake up dammit!"

"...Huh?" said Brandon again. "The mook are you talking about?"

Chad yanked open the curtains. "Look!"

The siren had been coming fast but now it abruptly blipped off. Brandon stared out the window: across the street were two cop cars and an idling fire truck. An ambulance had just arrived, and a crowd

304

was slowly gathering -- neighbors in bathrobes, kids on skates, middle-aged joggers, surfers on bikes -- while cops were stringing yellow tape along the cliffside railings. Brandon saw Troy in gym shorts and sneaks, his muscular body shiny with sweat.

"What happened, Chad?"

"One of your guests checked out last night... the endless out, if you get my drift."

"...What!"

Rex appeared in the doorway, in boxer shorts and rubbing his eyes. "What happened?"

"Get out!" snapped Chad, then added, "Sorry. Go make some coffee... you know how?"

"...Okay," said Rex, looking bewildered.

"What's going on?" Brandon demanded. "The party was totally boss, Chad!"

"Apparently not for everyone."

Brandon turned back to the window. A rope had been strung from the fire truck over the edge of the cliff, and a pair of firemen appeared carrying a rescue basket. A blanket-wrapped figure lay inside, and paramedics hurried to help.

Tommy burst puffing into the room, wearing only cutoffs. "I think it's Jason!"

"Jason?" Brandon faced Chad. "But, he didn't come to the party."

"So, why was he dressed in fur like one of your mutant characters?"

Brandon scrambled out of bed, but Chad grabbed his arm.

"Don't go out there! You either, Tommy! The cops could be at the door any minute! You better get your stories straight!"

"Zot?" said Tommy.

"The mook are you talking about?" yelled Brandon.

"Both of you sit," ordered Chad. "Now! ...What did Rex see?"

Brandon sat down on the bed beside Tommy. "There wasn't anything *to* see. ...Nothing bad, anyway."

Tommy added, "Rex fell asleep around eleven."

"Yeah," said Brandon. "We put him to bed in the guest room. As far as I know he's been there all night." He turned to the window again. "But, Jason didn't come to the party."

"Then why was he here?" asked Chad.

"I just told you..."

Chad pointed out the window. "I'll rephrase the question, why is he there?"

"How do you know it's him?" asked Brandon.

"Troy came running over when I was pulling into the driveway. He was jogging down to the Point. Said he stumbled and fell by the rails. That's when he saw Jason; recognized him from school."

Brandon stared out the window again as the... body... was transferred onto a gurney and loaded into the ambulance. A TV van rolled up.

Chad went on, "Troy called 911."

Tommy asked, "You saying Jason fell off the cliff?"

"It's pretty hard to fall over those rails... and let's assume in this neighborhood he probably wasn't pushed."

"You saying he jumped?" asked Brandon.

"I'm asking you two what happened last night... and you better tell me the truth."

"But it's only about thirty feet," said Brandon.

"To the rocks," said Chad. "He could have smashed his skull. Troy said there was a lot of blood."

"He was in fur?" asked Tommy.

"Like your Beastworld stuff."

"...So, he really wanted to come," said Brandon.

"Maybe that was him?" said Tommy. "Looking through the fence last night."

"But, he couldn't do it," said Brandon. "He couldn't come in and join us. ...He couldn't admit he was fat and have fun."

Chad frowned. "Nobody kills themselves 'cause they're fat."

"Yeah they do," said Brandon. "When they can't take the hate anymore."

"But you invited him to your party. Obviously you didn't hate him."

Tommy shook his head. "It was too little, too late. ...They can blame his death on 'obesity,' but not for the reasons they want."

Chad frowned again. "This isn't the time for moralizing. ...So he wasn't at your party at all?"

"No," said Brandon, picturing Jason lurking lonely outside in the dark, listening to other kids having fun but hating himself too much to join them because he'd been taught to hate himself. Just like he'd done on the websites. And every day at school.

"You trust your new friends?" asked Chad. "Like old-time spit-on-your-cut trust?"

"Yeah," said Brandon. "...But, what do you mean?" He looked out the window again; the ambulance was driving away, no need to use its siren. A man in a suit -- a police detective? -- had a note pad out and was talking to Troy. "Nobody had anything to do with... whatever happened out there."

"The cops might take a different view. ...You had a party last night," said Chad. "Everyone dressed like animals. And almost everybody was fat. Jason was fat and wearing fur. And now he's dead."

"Shit!" said Tommy.

"Ya think?" said Chad. "Who else knew about your party? Anybody at school?"

"Probably not," said Brandon.

"Probably might not be good enough. As mom would say, the evidence could be very damming."

Tommy asked, "Should we call everybody who came last night and tell 'em what happened?"

"Should we, Chad?" asked Brandon. "Get our story straight, like you said?"

"No," said Chad. "The cops could track the calls. Same if you messaged, texted or emailed, which would be worse 'cause they'd know what you said. And they could break a made-up story; question everyone separately."

"But, there isn't a story," said Brandon. "So, maybe the truth is the best defense?"

Chad snorted. "Which isn't much in a land of lies."

Brandon looked out the window again: most of the people had left by now, the kids on skates, the surfers on bikes, the bathrobed

307

neighbors and middle-aged joggers. The fire truck was pulling away, trailed by one of the cop cars. The TV crew was camming the cliff; and a talking-head woman, a Hollywood clone, was standing with a microphone, maybe waiting to interview Troy.

"Listen," said Chad. "*Carefully*. The worst-case scenario is, the cops find out about the party and try to blame Jason's death on you. ...Would you call Jason depressed?"

"A textbook case," said Tommy.

Brandon added, "It wasn't enough he got hated, he helped the haters hate him because he'd been taught he deserved to be hated."

"I might understand that," said Chad. "I've learned a little about the fat world since I seem to be getting a chubby brother. But I don't think the cops will. ...Think Jason did it on purpose? Right across the street like that? Maybe for payback on you?"

Brandon remembered the ice cream shop. He wished he'd tried to help Jason... wished he'd known *how* to help. "I don't think he'd do that. I guess it was just the closest place. Like, there he was, dressed for the party, but he couldn't make himself come in. Then there was nowhere else to go."

"You think he told his parents he was going to your party?"

"He only had a mom," said Tommy. "And I don't think he talked to her much. She was probably part of the reason he did it."

"I know you're smart," said Chad. "But, typical teenage American stupid is gonna play better right now."

"But I'm only twelve."

"That's good, keep practicing." Chad turned to Brandon. "Same goes for you. *We* know why Jason killed himself, let the experts figure it out."

"If they do they won't admit it," said Tommy.

"Remember you're only twelve," said Chad.

Brandon looked out the window again: the talking-head was talking to Troy. Brandon had a stupid thought; Troy should be making the most of this moment, showing off his Hollywood bod, but he only looked exhausted.

"Um..." said Rex from the doorway. "The coffee's ready. What happened?"

"Let's adjourn to the kitchen," said Chad. "And plan for damage control."

"Look!" cried Tommy.

Troy lay on the jogging path. A cop was giving him CPR. The talking-head was facing the camera... another teenage tragedy.

THIRTY-SIX

onald McDonald was on the TV dancing around like a moron on meth, surrounded by skinny, hyper kids all singing about how healthy it was to go out and play for an hour every day... preferably in McDonald Land.

"Shut that shit off!" muttered Troy.

Brandon thumbed the remote. "But exercise is healthy for you."

"Bite me, dork."

The hospital had ridiculous rooms as if designed by Dr. Seuss. They were barely the size of Brandon's closet, with tall narrow windows like prison cells, and were strangely shaped instead of square. Naturally the beds didn't fit, painfully wedged into odd-angled corners. The tiny space was made even smaller by a clumsy crank-up feeding table and an uncomfortable visitors chair that seemed to hate being sat on. The colors were mostly shades of purple, maybe intended to soothe troubled minds, though Brandon thought of funeral flowers and cards that read, *So sorry for your loss*.

Troy had lost his femmy gown, and Brandon had brought him a pair of boxers. He lay bare to the waist like the world's perfect boy... the Hollywood version, anyway. A plastic bag labeled, Patient's Belongings, lay at the foot of his bed, though only containing his gym shorts and worn out pair of running sneaks.

Brandon looked up at a chrome-plated pole that held a clear plastic bladder. A tube ran down to a needle taped in the back of Troy's left hand, and some sort of nourishment solution was dripping down the tube into Troy. "Taste good, man?"

"What about bite me don't you understand. ...And lunch sucked," added Troy. "Looked like somebody ate it already and

310

tasted even worse."

Brandon glanced at a spotless plate. "Looks like you ate it again anyhow."

"Hey, I was hungry. But if that was supposed to healthy food, I'd rather eat a stool sample."

Brandon laughed. "If it tastes like shit, it's gotta be healthy. But the doctor said you're supposed to eat. *Real* food for a change."

"Don't be cold, man, I almost died."

"I won't say I told you so. Your mom gave me the 411; she's been worried about you all summer since you got so 'healthy.' Between not eating actual food, popping those assoholic pills, running like some-thing was after your ass, and making love to those retarded weights, you could have been a healthy corpse."

"Thanks for not saying I told you so." Troy lay a hand on his chest and glanced at a blipping monitor. "They said I almost burned out my heart."

"What heart? But it's gonna be okay, isn't it?"

"They said there shouldn't be permanent damage. Not at my age anyway. But I can't play sports for the rest of the year, and I'm not supposed to run."

"Hey you get to be Special."

"I guess those dudes are cool."

"You know they are, I'm Special."

"Nah, you're just retarded... but you're special to me."

"Aw, let's kiss."

"My ass," said Troy. "They said I should gain some weight; my body doesn't have any reserves."

Brandon jiggled his belly. "I have lots of reserves."

"But how do you feel?"

"Like a happy beast. How do you feel?"

"Like a dog that got run over. But, are you gonna get fat?"

"By health-nazi standards I'm already obese."

"Nah, you're just chubby," said Troy, reaching to bobble Brandon's belly. "And you look kinda cool. But you know what I mean."

"I'm not a gainer, for me fat just happens. Like what happened to

Bosco I guess in the best summer of his life."

"I don't understand that gainer stuff, but Bosco looks boss," said Troy. "I always thought he did, but I couldn't admit it."

"Gaining or losing or..." Brandon poked one of Troy's stony pecs. "Muscle-building, is all about body-image. Whatever shape you're hap-py being. Or think you'd be happy being."

"And you like being chubby?"

Brandon shrugged. "I'm not obsessed with how I look, or how I'm being *told* to look by people who know what 'best' for me. There's good and bad about lots of things. Too much of something can make you unhappy just like having too little." He patted his chest. "This is my home in this time and place, but it's not a temple to anyone's god, including the hateful new god of 'health.'"

He glanced at a cross on the wall depicting a skinny and suffering Christ... the hospital was Catholic. "People aren't worshipping Him anymore, or whoever they think He is; instead they're worshipping their bodies. And they've started a new holy war against anybody who won't."

"And you're an unbeliever," said Troy, "so you're gonna get hated. But why make life harder than it already is?"

Brandon smiled. "I could kick you when you're down. You worked really hard to put yourself here."

"Yeah. But you won't 'cause you're cool."

Brandon considered. "Life hasn't been hard for me at all. Maybe that's one of my problems."

"So, you wanna get fat to make it harder?"

"I want to be me," said Brandon. "I'm not sure who that is yet, but I have some good friends who like who I am and maybe who I'm gonna be." He gently punched Troy's shoulder. "Including a friend I thought I lost."

"I'm back," said Troy. "Ta-da. ...Too bad about Jason, huh?"

"Yeah."

"You going to his funeral?"

"His mom isn't having one. Maybe she doesn't want people to see a fat kid in a coffin. Like, maybe they'll blame it on her."

"They should blame her because he's dead, but not because he was fat."

Brandon looked out the window, which overlooked a cemetery... not the healthiest view for a hospital. "And maybe they should blame the school for brainwashing kids to be 'healthy' instead of how to think for themselves. And all the people who hated on him. And all the anti-obesity shit, the junk science studies and 'clinical research'... nobody ever asks *whose* clinic... the jokes on TV and the internet rants, that made it okay to hate him."

Troy considered that and nodded. "Guess I let my mind get flabby with all that obsessing about my bod."

"All it needs is exercise; and a healthy mind doesn't hate."

"Did the cops find out about your party?"

"They never investigated," said Brandon. "Jason left a note. He scratched it on the railings with a piece of broken glass."

Brandon unfolded a newspaper clipping and handed it to Troy. "They said he was depressed because of his 'obesity'... but of course they wouldn't say *why*. It wouldn't have proved what they want to prove. Being fat didn't make him depressed and lead to suicide; being hated did. And that's what they won't admit. Jason was only collateral damage in the war on childhood obesity. Like a lot of other kids being hated just because of their weight. Most of them won't kill themselves, but they'll still be scarred for the rest of their lives. Like, somewhere inside they'll always be angry... sad, depressed or something un-healthy... that somebody mooked up their childhoods and wouldn't let them be happy kids."

"But others might be happy," said Troy. "That their parents or somebody else wanted them to lose weight."

Brandon nodded. "One size never fits all. What's wrong is trying to *make* it fit and hating anybody it doesn't." He glanced around the Dr. Suess room. "Like the Star-bellied Sneeches."

Troy read the clipping. "'Not to die but to be reborn, away from lands all tattered and torn.' That's Jimi Hendrix."

"Yeah," said Brandon, thinking that could have described what he'd felt out beyond the breakers.

"Jason was into Jimi," said Troy. "Who woulda thought?"

"That what's killed him. ...Nobody thought. Maybe he was kinda cool... knew about aliens and listened to Jimi... but all people thought about was his fat."

"Guess I haven't been thinking much, either."

Brandon smiled. "You said that already. I'm sure we can get your brain back in shape. ...By the way, did you see God?"

"Zot?"

"When you were on the other side?"

"Guess I didn't get that far. The last thing I remember seeing was some dude on a surfboard out on the ocean."

"Oh well," said Brandon. "Maybe next time."

"Cheer me up, dork. ...I didn't know you were religious."

"Let's say I met a tiki god out beyond the breakers."

"Did he tell you the answer is 42?"

"I won't know the answer until I get there. But then I won't need to ask the question."

"So, you got a girlfriend. ...Finally?"

"Had lunch with her today at the mall. By the way she's black. And fat both ways."

"Hey, you think I'm prejudiced?"

"You just got a little brainwashed. 'Course, there wasn't much to wash. ...Oh, I got you something." Brandon gave Troy a brown paper bag.

"*Playboy*, cool!"

"I was hoping you'd like it better than Muscle-boys In Baby Oil. Is it okay if you get sprung?"

"Too late to worry about it," said Troy, eagerly flipping pages. "Sweet centerfold! I'll save her for later."

"Don't blow another fuse. ...And you might need this," Brandon added, pulling out his wallet.

"When did you start packing rubbers?" asked Troy.

"When I thought I might need one... call it growing up a little."

"What should I do with it after?"

"There's a bio-hazard bag. ...How long are you gonna be in here?"

"They said about a week. Till my fluids get stable or something. Can you help with my homework? I don't wanna get behind."

"If you kiss my behind."

314

"Looks too much like your face."

"S'up, dudes?" asked Tommy, jiggling in from the hall.

"Hey, phat-boy," said Troy.

"He's baaaa-ak." Tommy flipped a switch on the monitor. "Woah, check it out, your heart stopped again."

"Mook!" yelled Troy.

A nurse hurried in.

Tommy switched the monitor on. "He was havin' a near-death experience seeing chubby cherubs."

"Don't play with that!" snapped the nurse. "And you should lose weight, you're obese!"

"Nah, I'm just fat. And I have better manners than you."

Troy added, "You could use a few pounds where it matters."

The nurse flushed, but glared at Tommy. "Are you family? No visitors except family."

"They're my brothers," said Troy. "My boss phat brothers." He pulled Tommy close. "Gimmie a hug."

"Help, I'm being molested!"

The nurse looked doubtful but left.

"Don't you think that was gay?" asked Tommy.

Troy flipped open the magazine. "I still like her tits better than yours."

"Woah! So do I!"

Troy sniffed the air. "What smells good?"

"My dick," said Tommy. He plopped a McDonald's bag on the table. "I brought you a super-size Happy Meal and I didn't even spit on it."

"Thanks," said Troy. "I'm starving."

THIRTY-SEVEN

Summer happened before Brandon knew it.

It had seemed like light-years away in those long dark months after Christmas when rain hissed over the patio and the ocean crashed against the cliffs, spewing spray across the street that rattled his window glass. But, time did go faster as you got older, flinging the future into your face before you knew the past was gone.

The present time was early June, close to midnight on the last day of school, and this had been the best party yet, topping even New Year's Eve and the feast of the beasts that had rocked Spring Break... which Bosco called Easter Vacation. Brandon had just kissed Darla goodnight, both lingering long in each other's arms until the bus driver tapped his horn. Brandon waved as the bus drove away, and Darla blew him a kiss from a window. A car rolled by and somebody yelled, "Put a shirt on, fatty!"

Brandon flipped a finger and waited, but the car kept going toward Lighthouse Point. Then he returned to his driveway to say goodbye to his other friends, Carlos, Danny, Zach, and Rex, all of whom had come with dates.

Carlos and Danny were still fat boys, proud of their heritage and proud of themselves. Zach and Nikki still had feeding sessions, and Zack now looked about nine months pregnant. Rex had gained almost thirty pounds, but also a sudden six vertical inches.

All the beasts got A's in P.E. thanks to Danny Little-Wing, and despite Coach's rants that fat kids were failures.

Travis, Brandon, Bosco and Rex had aced Creative Writing class. Brandon and Travis's *The Time Surfer-boy* was published in the school magazine and won the Best Story Award. Travis had used his graphic skills to illustrate Brandon's Beastworld book with furry, big-eyed characters of every size and color, and Mr. Akida's agent was shopping it around. Brandon and Travis were collaborating on *The Adventures Of A Quarter-Ton Kid.*

Chad had taken Brandon's side to stay in public school, but Brandon had decided not to. Spending a year in public school had been like going to survival camp and learning how to live in a world of ignorance and conformity where thinking was a handicap. The system was geared to crank out clones... lean, mean, unthinking zombies, physically fit for work or war, who never questioned their televised orders to buy and consume everything on the planet and hate anyone they were told to hate.

And zombies ate brains of those who still had them.

Chad had been right last fall; about throwing away a good education just to have "regular friends." But they would always be his friends no matter what school he went to. Real friends were forever, and they came in all colors and sizes.

And maybe he'd been right himself, that most of the things that mattered in life would happen somewhere between skateboards and wheelchairs, between rock concerts and hearing aids, between beer-bongs and Ben-Gay for arthritis, and he should be thinking of them. A private high school offered scholarships, and Travis would easily qualify, so he and Brandon could go together.

Brandon glanced across the street, seeing a pair of rolly shadows hand-in-hand by the moonlit sea. Tommy was walking Terri home, and not for exercise. Tommy's weight had stabilized after winning his diet wars; he skated, swam, and had learned to surf, right along with Ro.

A few days after Jason's death a city maintenance truck had rolled up and a man had painted the railing where Jason had left his last words... a neighbor complained it was morbid. At the start of each party since Halloween the beasts all gathered on the cliff and an offering of pizza and beer was solemnly thrown to the sea. Maybe Jason had jumped to the alternate future that caught the right wave in the past?

The house's front door was open, and Ronny and Donny came

waddling out to clamber into their mom's minivan. The twins hadn't lost any weight, but months of swimming in Brandon's pool, and casual hikes behind their house had strengthened their muscles a lot. They did more of what they wanted to do and checked out things they'd thought they couldn't. There had also been trips to Bosco's beach... a timeless hate-free zone.

The summer night was clear and warm. The party had been amphibious, and Brandon wore only his cutoff jeans, ragged and tight with three buttons open, his belly lolling over in front. His boy-breasts bobbed as he crossed the lawn, displaying their innie nipples. The light from the doorway darkened a bit as Travis, Kelvin and Ro emerged, also wearing cutoffs. Kelvin was as ripped as ever, a midnight mutant panther prince. Travis and Ro hadn't gained much weight, but both looked naked in frontal view. They also swam in Brandon's pool and hiked the Boardwalk beach every morning. The haters had learned to leave them in peace... hating wasn't as fun when the hated fought back.

"Boss party," said Kelvin.

"Bitchin'," said Ro.

"Phat," said Travis.

Their father's van rolled up to the curb, displaying its happy fat boy graphic, and Travis gave Ro a blubbery hug. "Go with Kel, I'll catch a bus."

"Where's Bosco?" asked Brandon, joining Travis on the porch.

"Still talking with Troy about surfing."

"Got time for another beer?" asked Brandon.

"Always time for beer," said Travis, subsiding massively onto the step. "The ocean looks pretty, let's have it out here."

Brandon went into the living room as Troy came up the hall. Troy was also in cutoffs, and toting two longnecks of Bud. He'd filled out a lot this winter, adding mass to his muscles.

"Brought these for you and Travis," said Troy, handing Brandon the bottles.

"You started reading minds?" asked Brandon.

"I know yours like a pre-school book."

"What's up with Bosco?" asked Brandon. "He's been kinda quiet

318

tonight."

"I noticed," said Troy. "Like he's not all here. I'd think he was slammed, but he never gets slammed."

"He's probably got summer surf on his mind. Wanna stay for another beer?"

"Thanks, but I better get to bed. I'm not supposed to be up this late. Doctor's orders. He'd shit granola and carrot sticks if he knew I was drinking and surfing with you, but I feel a lot better than when I was 'healthy.'"

"So, how are you doing?" asked Brandon. "Now that you got a heart again, not to mention a brain of your own."

"Guess all I need now is some courage."

"Hey that's a good one."

"The tests look good," said Troy. "But I'm still gonna take it easy this summer. I'm selling my weights; I need a new wetsuit since I gained a few."

"What about running the race?"

"Nobody ever wins it, no matter what shape they're in." Troy looked out at the moon-sparkled sea. "Money and toys don't count over there. And, assuming there is a God, your soul isn't judged by BMI. ...You doing anything tomorrow? We could skate down to the Boardwalk, get a burger and play some games."

"Sure," said Brandon. "And maybe you'll finally meet a girl."

"Thanks, I needed that."

"So, you're up for skating again?"

"No trick moves, but I'm phat."

Brandon gave Troy a hug. "Yeah, you are. See you tomorrow."

"May all your dreams be wet."

Brandon went out, sat down next to Travis and gave him one of the bottles.

"Thanks, Bosco," said Travis.

"Zot?"

"Oh," said Travis. "Guess I was lost in space." He studied Brandon a moment. "Maybe I didn't notice 'cause I see you every day, but you and Bosco could be twins since you joined the chubby club." Then he gripped his bottle cap. "Houston, we have a

319

problem."

"Zot?"

"It's not a twist-off, Bosco brought these."

"Beans." Brandon checked his own bottle. "They *can't* be from 1963. Maybe they're from Mexico."

"You need a logical explanation?"

"Some of our readers might."

"Boss party, Brandy-buck." Bosco ambled out of the house, cigar in one hand, a beer in the other, his ragged cutoffs riding low.

"Thanks," said Brandon. "Got an opener?"

"Never without one, dude." Bosco opened the bottles with his Cub Scout knife — won, he'd said, in a poker game -- and plopped down on the porch.

Travis took a sip. "Tastes as fresh as yesterday."

"Just got 'em yesterday," said Bosco.

Brandon laughed. "Which yesterday?"

"The regular kind; the one whose today was tomorrow," said Bosco.

He pulled two more cigars from a pocket and fired them with a wooden match. The boys sat smoking in silence a while, sipping beer, gazing out at the ocean. The moonlight seemed to make a path that might have led to the past or the future... or maybe just to *there*. "You dudes seem kinda thinky tonight."

Travis smiled. "I was gonna say the same about you."

Brandon studied the moonlit path. "I've been thinking a lot... you have to choose the right wave to ride, and sometimes that isn't easy."

"Most of the time you can feel it," said Bosco. "An' trust the tikis if you can't." He dug in his cutoffs again and pulled out a pair of necklaces. "Here, dudes, I made 'em for you."

"Yesterday, no doubt," said Travis, putting on the necklace.

"The right yesterday," said Brandon, slipping his god around his neck. "The one that earned the right tomorrow."

"There's only one today," said Bosco. "An' that's what you gotta get right for tomorrow." He glanced at the rusty Volkswagen van sitting in the driveway. A pair of long-boards were strapped to its roof.

"Hate to say it, dudes, but this is goodbye till we meet again."

"...Oh," said Brandon. "Going on safari?"

"Waves to ride, beer to drink, burgers to scarf on the beach. So much time an' so much to do. You know how that is. Heh."

The van's windshield was like a mirror, and Brandon saw two chubby blond boys sitting beside a young black Buddha. The image was reversed, and for a moment he wasn't sure who was Bosco and who was himself, especially now with the necklace. "We'll miss you, man."

"A lot of people will," said Travis. "Even if they don't know what they're missing."

"Here's the key to the beach," said Bosco. "Surf there any time."

END

ABOUT THE AUTHOR

Jess Mowry was born in 1960 near Starkville, Mississippi. When he was only a few months old his father took him to live in Oakland, California. Mowry's father was a voracious reader who introduced his son to books at a very early age. Jess attended a public school, but despite his love of reading, dropped out at age thirteen, part way through the eighth grade and worked with his father in the scrap-iron business. In his late teens, Jess moved to Arizona to work as a truck driver and heavy equipment operator. He also lived and worked in Alaska as an engineer aboard a tugboat and as an aircraft mechanic on Douglas C-47 cargo planes, as well as at a children's refuge in Haiti.

Mowry has written twenty-five books and many short stories about black children and teens in a variety of genres, ranging from inner-city settings to the forests of Haiti, the wilds of Alaska, the Arizona desert, the Caribbean Sea, and the African veldt. While some of his novels are set in Oakland and deal with social issues, such as poverty, violence, drugs, gangs, teenage sexuality, and school drop-outs, Mowry has also written ghost tales, as well as novels featuring Voodoo and African magic, in addition to sea stories, and compiled an anthology of Victorian ghost stories.

Jess Mowry lives in Oakland, California.

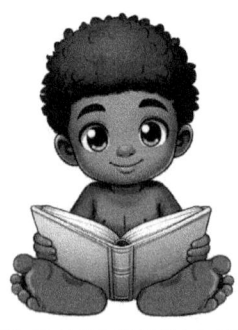

THIS BOOK IS ALSO AVAILABLE IN A KINDLE EDITION

322

OTHER ANUBIS BOOKS

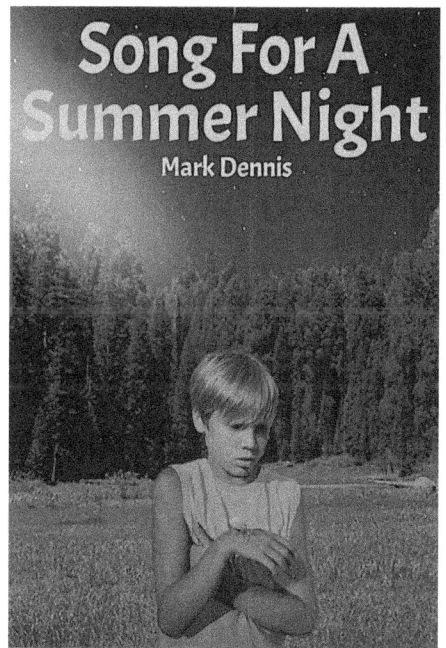

AVAILABLE ON AMAZON

www.ingramcontent.com/pod-product-compliance
Lightning Source LLC
Chambersburg PA
CBHW071530260626
47170CB00002B/577